C is for CONQUER

Advance Praise for

C is for CONQUER

"Bobbi's book chronicles her amazing story through a heartfelt, down-to-Earth voice that we can all relate to. What she has endured and, most importantly, bounced back from, makes for an inspiring tale worth sharing regardless of your personal life experiences. I have known Bobbi personally for a decade at the time of this review and shared in her mission through various community projects. She is an inspiring, fun-loving and authentic person that is out to create change in an increasingly important area for our youth. Her story illustrates these qualities colorfully and I highly recommend it to anyone."

—**Tudor Alexander**, author, speaker, entrepreneur

"Wow! What a trip! Bobbi's honest, sincere and detailed way of describing what she went through and how she felt about it, dealt with it emotionally, and analyzed it was amazing. Bobbi's sense of humor throughout delights. I now have a reference to share with anyone going through the cancer journey to help them on the way through and coming home again to healing and definitely thriving."

—**Carol E. Becker**, CCht, Dementia Therapy Specialist, Master NLP TimeLine® Practitioner, Trauma Therapist

"Holy cow… the death of a child, death of a sister and then CANCER! You Bobbi, are a bright star. Thank you for opening your heart, your soul and sharing the raw details of your journey and how you embraced the lessons that came with your diagnosis. You really never know until you know; the devastating side effects of cancer treatment, the emotional toll it takes and the spiritual gifts that come from your healing.

Bobbi reminds us the importance of research, advocating for yourself, the power of natural healing and how stress kills! She graciously and with humor gives you a birds eye view of how a cancer diagnosis suddenly fills your life with doctor appointments, scans, lab work and then collateral damage. Through example, she reminds us the gift of relationships and the value of accepting help. This book is full of great tips, don't wait until after treatment. Read it now!"

—**Edna Ness**, Best-selling author: *Radical Recovery,*
Extraordinary Healing with Oxygen
and Light after Chemo and Radiation

C is for
CONQUER
Moving From Surviving
to THRIVING

Bobbi Lynn Sudberry

NEW YORK

LONDON • NASHVILLE • MELBOURNE • VANCOUVER

C is for CONQUER
Moving From Surviving to THRIVING

Published in New York, New York, by Morgan James Publishing. Morgan James is a trademark of Morgan James, LLC. www.MorganJamesPublishing.com

ISBN 978-1-64279-343-7 paperback
ISBN 978-1-64279-344-4 eBook
ISBN 978-1-64279-345-1 hardcover
Library of Congress Control Number: 2018913163

Cover Design by:
Rachel Lopez
www.r2cdesign.com

Interior Design by:
Bonnie Bushman
The Whole Caboodle Graphic Design

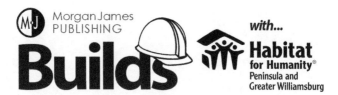

In an effort to support local communities, raise awareness and funds, Morgan James Publishing donates a percentage of all book sales for the life of each book to Habitat for Humanity Peninsula and Greater Williamsburg.

Get involved today! Visit
www.MorganJamesBuilds.com

To Ric and my Children
True Unconditional Love

Table of Contents

Foreword

Bobbi Lynn Sudberry and I met in December of 2010 in New York City at an event called It's Time to Talk: a day devoted to talking about domestic and teen dating violence. Bobbi was there on behalf of Kaity's Way, a nonprofit organization she founded with her husband, Ric, after an ex-boyfriend tragically murdered their daughter, Kaity, during her senior year of high school in January of 2008. I was at the event as an author and a survivor of teen dating violence, and the juxtaposition of my experience and Kaity's was humbling. Looking into Bobbi's eyes, I knew that Kaity's story had nearly been my own. My role at It's Time to Talk was that of the victim turned survivor while Bobbi's was that of a grieving mother, each galvanized by the notion that our collective experiences could prevent others from falling prey to an abusive person.

As if wading through the waters of unspeakable grief wasn't enough, in August of 2009, the universe handed Bobbi another life to advocate for—her own—when she learned she had cancer. In a style all her own, Bobbi has chronicled her journey as a survivor of breast cancer, but different from other self-help books, *C is for Conquer* makes the reader feel as if they are sitting with Bobbi in the quiet of a cozy room listening to her remarkable story of survival over a cup of tea. From candid descriptions of her diagnosis, treatments, and recovery, Bobbi shows that the battle with cancer is one she was prepared to win. The lessons Bobbi learns are many, but the one that resonates almost as if a gift is that even with the grief she carries, hers is a life worth living.

In many respects, Bobbi is the phoenix that rises from the ashes—ashes of despair and ashes of surgeries, chemotherapy, and radiation. She rises with newfound clarity about how she wants to conduct her life, choose her words, and peel back the shell of defensiveness. Bobbi's new lease on life allows her the freedom to be the best version of herself—a helper—something I surmise we could all use a lot more of: people dedicated to making the world a better place one person and one moment at a time.

—**Elin Stebbins Waldal**, Author of the award-winning book,
*Tornado Warning, a Memoir of Teen Dating Violence
and its Effect on a Woman's Life,* Freeland, Washington

Preface

This book was written with the best of intentions in mind. It is my hope that someone who has had a rough go at it in one way or another realizes they are not alone. Not to mention realizing that things happen, and it is futile to try to control anything or anyone beyond your own self. If we were able to control those things, you can be darn sure things would have been vastly different in my life.

At times my emotions can be very raw, and anger is apparent. Please know this book is in no way meant to hurt or offend anyone intentionally or unintentionally. It is simply an account and expression of my feelings while on a journey not of my choosing. There is no need to read between the lines or assume anything about what I say. I say what I say because I chose to say it. How I say it is how it is meant to be heard and understood. You may also notice I create words of my own to describe things. I do this because I can. Anyone can and if it makes them feel good and it doesn't hurt anyone, they should. I publicly speak about my trials and tribulations to simply inspire and educate others, as it is my belief that we exist to be happy helping ourselves as well as others.

"And just as the Phoenix rose from the ashes, she too will rise. Returning from the flames, clothed in nothing but her strength, more beautiful than ever before."

—Shannen Heartzs

Acknowledgements

Ric Sudberry: you love me so unconditionally and showed me what true love really is, for which I am eternally grateful.

My children: I appreciate your help and patience with me while on this journey. It wasn't easy for me, so I know it must have been a challenge for you.

Dione Lathrop: your friendship, fun times, and help with the editing of this book is greatly appreciated and will never be forgotten.

Janie Saurette: for loving me all my life despite me being the reason you don't like mustard.

Elin Stebbins Waldal: for allowing me to learn from your experience as well as your honesty. Timing is of the essence and you certainly helped with that.

Chief Jerald Monahan: Thank you so very much for introducing me to Morgan James Publishing. I commend your service not only in law enforcement but your continued efforts to help others and put an end to domestic violence.

Morgan James Publishing team: you saw this diamond in the rough and have been so gracious to share your expertise to help me to polish it and share it with the world. Your constant encouragement and empowerment while on this journey has been absolutely inspiring for me. Your patience, dedication, and faith in me has been extraordinary and more than I can ever imagine or wish for.

Everyone mentioned in this book: Thank you from the bottom of my heart.

God Bless you all!

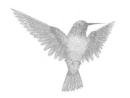

Chapter 1

That's Not Right

I t was a very hot and muggy evening August 12, 2009. I launched into my daily routine when I got home from work. I changed into my favorite bright yellow, colorful, lightweight house dress I bought when we vacationed in Rocky Point, Mexico in 2004. The memories of that vacation with the kids and my sister, Christy, and her kids made me feel good. At that time in my life, I needed all the good feelings I could muster up. No bra of course and my thick, medium-length, platinum over dark auburn hair was pulled back into a ponytail at the crown of my head. This was my let-it-all-hang-out mode. I headed to the computer room to prepare myself for a conference I am scheduled to attend in about a week and a half on behalf of Kaity's Way, the non-profit organization I co-founded with my husband. In addition to working full-time as an Operations Supervisor for a company that coordinates home health care for patients, I had voluntarily taken on a mission through Kaity's Way. Kaity's Way is my passion, but the full-time job paid the bills.

As I rose from my desk to retrieve my briefcase, the inside of my upper right arm brushed against my right breast and I felt something odd that stopped me dead in my tracks. So, I poked around the upper right quadrant of my right breast and thought to myself, "That's not right." I felt a lump the size of a quarter. "Okay, it is too late to call my physician, so I will call her tomorrow." I went back to getting ready for the conference, but looking back, how was it that I was able to feel something the size of a quarter as deep in my breast as it was? Weird, right?

Don't get me wrong, this was concerning, but the previous years had been a series of very unfortunate events for my family, so I guess I was somewhat desensitized and figured things just couldn't get any worse …

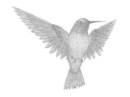

Chapter 2

Painful Times

The absolute worst part of the previous years happened on January 28, 2008. Our 17-year-old daughter, Kaity, on her way home from school, was murdered by her ex-boyfriend. Kaity was a beautiful young lady who had her whole life ahead of her. She was a senior in her last semester of high school. Kaity was very intelligent and had been accepted to Northern Arizona University, where she was looking forward to studying wildlife sciences.

This ripped us to shreds. As a family we remained steadfast, but inside each of us a hole had been drilled, never to heal over or close. What we knew as normal no longer existed. To this day it still feels like a very bad nightmare we cannot seem to wake from.

Kaity's older brothers had to be flown in from Florida and Illinois. Her younger sister still lived at home with us and was present when the devastating news of Kaity's passing was delivered to us. Her older sister lived about 20 miles west of Phoenix. Family and very dear friends without hesitation came to our sides to comfort and support us. My sister Lorie, who had recently lived with us off and on for a couple of years was very close to all of us, but she and Kaity had a special little bond as they were starting anew at the same time. Lorie jumped right in and fielded the media for us as we were barely capable of making the funeral arrangements. God bless her for taking on that role, as it could not have been easy for her by any means.

Lorie was also there for me when everyone inevitably had to go back to their lives. She saw the state I was in and made it a point to call me often and come by the house at least once a week, usually Wednesdays, to check on me. She chose Wednesdays because my husband worked the swing shift and was not home until 11:20pm. Lorie watched as I had gone from a very outgoing person to someone who didn't leave the house unless it was absolutely necessary. I would sit on the swing out front and look down the street, waiting for Kaity to come around the corner, as if she was on her way home from school. Lorie knew what I was doing, so she would come over and keep me company.

Lorie was a very bright spot at the time and I really looked forward to her visits. We would sit and talk about anything that came to mind; work, family issues, future, angels, what to do next. Often times she did most of the talking, but I was happy to listen and have her there. She never pushed me or got frustrated with me. Instead, she encouraged and empowered me. She also introduced me to the Four Agreements. At the time, I was not very receptive as I was still trying to figure out why Kaity was gone.

When Lorie and I were kids, we were your typical sisters. I was the serious, needed-to-be-perfect one and Lorie was truly a free spirit. She was the epitome of 'just do it and ask forgiveness later'. Lorie was witty, had a sharp tongue, and was absolutely brilliant. Sometimes we were close, other times not so close. Even so, I was very protective of her. No one messed with my little sister and when we were older, she would help me out when I needed it, especially when it came to the kids.

There was a period of about five years, 2001 to 2006, in which Lorie and I were not getting along at all. Lorie had battled with substance abuse since she was 16 years old. I believe within that time frame she was possibly very deep into the drug scene. I had become her nemesis because I was on a completely different track and we could not relate. I was raising a family, working full-time, and going to college; pre-pharmacy at the time. In late 2006, about the same time Kaity began her very first dating relationship, Lorie, at our mother's urging—or rather insistence—asked me if she could move into my house as she intended to end her on-again, off-again relationship with drugs. Mom and Lorie both knew we did not tolerate drugs under any circumstances in our household. I spoke with my husband. We discussed the possibilities but felt deep inside Lorie was absolutely serious about her goal to get clean and stay clean. It took a lot of guts for her to ask if she could come live with us considering the distance between she and I. We cautiously agreed to the arrangement and Lorie moved in with us and our two youngest daughters Kaity and Virginia (aka Mooki).

Incidentally, this was our mother's way of getting Lorie and I back into each other's lives. Chalk one up for mom here.

Allowing Lorie to move in with us was one of the best decisions we made. It took some time, but she really did it. Lorie kicked the drug habit! I had my sister back and our relationship flourished. Lorie's presence in the house had given our lives a whole new fun-filled dimension. Lorie had a life force like no other. She was still that free spirit. We had some great times while she lived with us. Her presence and mannerisms were so quirky at times that if you weren't falling out laughing because of something she said or did, at the very least she would put a smile on your face. I could go on forever about her, but that is another book I intend to write because life with Lorie was very eventful.

Brace yourself, because here we go with another really unfortunate event for our family. On June 9, 2009, I was at my day job and I received a frantic message from my mother. Something had happened to Lorie. I called my mother back and she told me she is not sure what happened, but a police officer called her and said Lorie passed away and was at John C. Lincoln Hospital off 3rd Street and Dunlap in Phoenix. What the fluff! I had just seen Lorie on Sunday. She looked tired, but seemed like she was okay. Immediately, I fell to my knees and began wailing. I went to the floor in disbelief. My co-workers and boss came to my aid and helped me get to my car. Lorie, 43 years old, had been found in her car, which was parked in front of a small strip mall in Phoenix. We would find out later the cause of death was undetermined, but foul play had been ruled out.

Once again, our family was in the throes of despair and it was everything we could do to keep it together. My mother was so angry, and I could relate. Lorie's kids; a 20-year-old son and two daughters, 16 and 17 years old, were shocked and beside themselves. It was incomprehensible to my brother and two other sisters. We hardly had time to come to terms with losing Kaity and now we had suddenly lost another wonderful person we loved. I remember when I called my husband to give him the bad news. I tried to keep my composure, but was not at all successful. I said to him, "Lorie was now dancing with Kaity in heaven." That was how I saw it then and still see it now. Those two had become so very close and without a doubt I am sure Kaity was there to welcome Lorie.

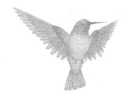

Chapter 3

What to Do?

At roughly 10:00 in the morning on the 13th of August I was at my day job trying to work up the courage to contact my family doctor. I was hemming and hawing around, but knew I needed to have the lump assessed. The thought that kept going through my mind was; How am I going to go see the doctor and not tell my husband? At least until I found out if there was really anything to worry about. I just didn't want to worry him needlessly. He is my best friend, so I am not one to lie or keep secrets from him. Given all we had been through in the last 20 months with losing Kaity and Lorie, I did not relish the idea of piling on with another issue.

This was where things got a little strange. As I was considering what to do I received a very random text message from our oldest daughter, Yvonne. The message said, "Mom, have you been to the doctor lately?" No kidding, seriously out of the blue that is what she asked me. Baffled by her question and given what I had been contemplating, I responded, "I was just fixin to make an appointment, why do you ask?" You may want to sit down for this next part, because her response said, "My friend told me you need to see your doctor because you have breast issues." As God or any other higher power is my witness, that conversation took place verbatim. Given my spiritual nature, I was on it! I immediately contacted my doctor's office and scheduled an appointment for August 14th first thing in the morning. I did tell my husband about the appointment that evening. I really didn't see any way around it and felt I needed his support either way.

The doctor confirmed what I was feeling was a lump and gave me a STAT prescription for a mammogram and ultrasound of my right breast. I scheduled the tests for August 19th and a follow-up visit with my doctor on the 21st of August. The results were suspicious to sum it up.

The ultrasound found there was "a multilobular hypoechoic mass with posterior acoustic shadowing in the 11:00 position of the breast, overall 2.6 x 2.1 cm in size. This correlated with an ill-defined abnormality on the mammogram." The radiologist's mammogram report said "**SUSPICIOUS OF MALIGNANCY**" exactly like that. In addition it said, "The 2.5cm x 2.5 cm irregular density in the right breast likely represents as a solid mass and appears suspicious of malignancy. A biopsy is recommended." At that point my husband insisted on being with me every step of the way as things progressed. My doctor gave me a referral to a surgeon to schedule a biopsy.

I had a conference to attend the following week and I was bound and determined not to miss it!

My first appointment with the surgeon was scheduled for August 31st. The surgeon reviewed the test results and agreed a biopsy was needed. 75 percent of the time the lumps are benign. The surgeon was trying to keep a positive attitude, but for some reason I could not comprehend what she was saying and so I questioned her. I am not sure how I came across, but she seemed to lose her patience with me for a moment and repeated herself in a tone like she was saying, "Snap out of it." The look on my husband's face was very guarded as he was trying to keep a positive attitude as well.

The biopsy was done in the surgeon's office on September 7th. My husband was so intent on being with me through this that the surgeon had to ask him to leave the room while she did the biopsy. My husband was a medical technician in the Air Force and tried to plead his case, but the surgeon was not about to give him any ground. She explained to me it was too unpredictable how someone would react to what she was about to do, and they did not need another patient to take care of while trying to take care of me. The biopsy was done and the follow-up visit was scheduled for September 14th.

As we were leaving the office, my dear husband was annoyed at the fact he could not be with me through the biopsy. This was sweet, because my husband usually didn't let most things bother him. He is a very roll-off-the-shoulder type of person, more so since losing Kaity.

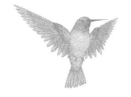

Chapter 4

Disbelief

O
n September 10th, I received a call from the surgeon's office. They had rescheduled my follow-up appointment for September 11th. I tried to remain positive but knew deep down that this was not a good sign. When we arrived at the surgeon's office we were immediately called to the back. When she came into the room I was sitting on the exam table and my husband was in a chair across the room. The surgeon tried to hide her emotions as she told us I had breast cancer. She seemed sincerely affected by the fact that she had to deliver such bad news to us and I genuinely felt bad for her. She knew by now what we had been through in the last 20 months and the last thing she wanted to do was add to it.

Upon receiving the news, keeping a stiff upper lip, I looked at her and said, "I got this doc, it's going to be okay, this is nothing compared to losing a child. I would have breast cancer befall me several times over if it meant we could have our daughter back." She knew I meant what I said and gave me a hug and went into the usual protocol. She referred me to the office case manager, who gave me a bunch of literature and scheduled the lumpectomy for September 17th.

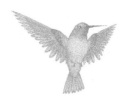

Chapter 5

Who and How
to Tell Them

My husband and I drove home in utter bewilderment. Once again, we were thrust into a journey we did not sign up for but somehow end up on. I remember I looked at my husband and for the last time I said with exasperation, "What's next?!"

He said, "Don't say that, it only opens the door for bad things to happen." Next, we discussed who we were going to tell, when, and how. We decided to start with the kids.

Yvonne would be the first of our children to be told. She is the oldest and the one who knew I was going to the doctor for breast issues. Then we would tell our youngest daughter, Virginia aka Mooki. We were not quite sure when we would tell Mooki. She had started down a dark path after losing her sister Kaity and was estranged from us at the time.

A few months earlier, Mooki had taken off with who she thought was a friend—we will call her TM for trouble maker—at the time to live somewhere else. In the midst of everything we had been through, losing Kaity, then Lorie, TM was a lingering dark spot. She was the true definition of a self-serving, manipulative leech who latched on to Mooki at a very vulnerable time in her life.

After Kaity passed, we tried to get help for Mooki. She refused counseling but I made her go with me one time and she would not open up. I took her for her own counseling sessions to no avail. We tried talking with her on several occasions but failed miserably. By this time, TM has Mooki believing she was the only one who understood and loved her. Where the heck do these people come from and why do they think they are so entitled? Mooki started sneaking out with TM and stopped coming home at a reasonable time. When we looked for Mooki and brought her home, she took off at the first opportunity she saw.

We dealt with this for several weeks and eventually decided to take a different approach. We found out the place she kept running to was stable and caring. So, essentially, we gave her some space. A few months later, Mooki agreed to come back home on the condition we let TM come too. TM gave us the woe-is-me story and presented as a poor soul that had been kicked out of her home by her family at 17 years old. To hear TM tell it, she did everything right, but no matter what she did her parents were the worst and would always put her down. We did concede to letting TM move in under the guise of her woe-is-me story, but to protect ourselves we had one of her parents write up an affidavit stating she had their permission to live with us. My guess was since she was going to be 18 years old within a couple of months, her parents may have figured, "what's the harm," and provided us with a letter of consent that they were okay with TM living with us. Our real reason for letting TM move in was because we saw through her bull and, with all the patience in the world, worked to expose it in such a way Mooki would see TM for who she really was. That was not to say we didn't hope TM would prove us wrong or at least turn over a new leaf.

For several months we tried to help TM get herself together. We supported her by giving her a roof over her head and food in her stomach; we gave her the necessary tools to get her GED and a job. All the while she did nothing but lie around and go out with her friends with Mooki in tow. She wouldn't even do chores we listed for her to do, which would have taken no more than 30 minutes a day to do. Eventually, we gave TM an ultimatum; she either started showing some effort to get her GED, a job and contribute to the household or she was going to have to leave. The next thing we knew, she and Mooki had left while we were at work. Apparently, TM was part of a lesson Mooki had to learn.

We elected not to tell our sons RJ and Dan until everything was over and I was cancer-free. As for the rest of the family, we would tell only my aunt at first. We would also tell Ric's mother, brother Cliff, and sister Angela. We would hold off on telling my mother due to the recent loss of Lorie and the fact that she was helping my youngest sister battle her own demons.

Quite honestly my mother had become so angry, for which I felt the brunt (or so it seemed that way), after losing Lorie. I was kind of afraid and not sure of what her reaction would be towards me. Mentally I was trying to be tough, but deep down I felt very fragile. Would she see this as small potatoes since she was so desensitized by what happened to Lorie? After all, she just lost a child also. Could she handle just one more issue with her grown children? It was way too much to consider what direction this would take!

Why not tell the boys? RJ was 23 years old, in the Air Force and was stationed in Korea at the time. He had nine months left on his assignment. My prognosis was not terminal therefore we believed it was unlikely RJ would be allowed to come back to the states. With this in mind, it seemed as though it would only hurt RJ if he were to know what was going on with me. We tried to put ourselves in his shoes. If one of our mothers were going through something similar, we would have wanted to be with them. Sensing RJ would feel the same way, could you imagine his disappointment when his commander told him, "Sorry your mom has cancer, but she is not terminal, so we cannot allow you to go home." I know that would not have sat well with me if I were in his shoes. RJ is mild mannered, but he had recently lost his sister and his aunt. Then to hear his mother has breast cancer … I feared this might push him just a little too far and possibly over the edge.

Dan was in a very different boat. He was 21 years old and still acting out due to the loss of his sister and he was also hurting over the loss of his aunt. His anger was very prevalent, and he had moved to Massachusetts in an effort to deal with his pain. We agreed telling Dan would do nothing more than add insult to injury.

Before telling anyone in the family I contacted my employer and let them know I had been diagnosed with breast cancer and would be taking a leave of absence. I made this decision because my aunt had battled breast cancer three years before and worked at the same time. It was a struggle for her, but she had only her income to live on. I decided I was going to put everything I had into beating this and that meant decreasing my level of stress immensely.

My job was very stressful as it was drilled into us constantly that patients depended on us to make sure they received the follow up care they needed at home. It was a 24 hour, seven day a week job that required us to be basically on call. When I had first started with this division, the work week averaged 60 to 70 hours for nearly two years. After losing Kaity, I scaled my hours back to no more than 50 hours a week. Nonetheless, the stressors were still there. Not only was the necessary patient care a stressor, but the office politics were ridiculous. The egos that permeated that place were overwhelming. Since losing Kaity, I had absolutely no ego. I had come to realize I had no control over anything but me and had become a very humble person. Ego just did not play into my life anymore. Looking back, I wished I had known to kick ego out of my life long before. Live and learn, right?

All in all, I had paid for short-term disability for many years and even bought up to receive 50 percent of my income if I were to need it. Now I needed it. Electing to go on disability did take our income down by nearly a third, but finances were the least of my worries. My health was much more important. If anything, I needed to prioritize what was really important in life and realize stress does not do anything or anybody any good.

My employer accepted me going out on disability and the Senior Project Coordinator, Kara, who was a very dear friend, did everything she could to get all the paperwork in order so that my disability would go smoothly. I cannot tell you what a help and relief it was to have had one less thing to worry about.

Later that evening we went over to my Aunt Janie's house and broke the news to her. She was the first because of our close relationship and her previous battle with breast cancer. It was so hard to tell her. I cried as I said the words, "I have breast cancer." Mostly, because of the pain I knew she would feel for me. Not to mention, I was sure it would bring up some agonizing memories for her. Janie took the news well, but I could see the concern in her eyes. I let her know we had not told my mother yet and we were not quite sure when we would.

When Janie went through breast cancer in 2006, I helped from a distance. Besides working what felt like a bazillion hours a week, I struggled with the idea of seeing this strong and seemingly invincible woman who knew me all my life in such a vulnerable state. My mother took care of her sister through her bout with cancer, then my cousins, Janie's children, Tammy and Chris, helped out when they could. I often asked if there was anything I could do, but my mom usually said they had things under control. I do remember when Janie had finished all her treatments; I went over to see her and ended up crying and apologizing for not being around more while she was sick. She said she had had enough help and there was no reason to apologize. There she was, someone who had gone to hades and back, bald as a cue ball consoling me. Her eyes were so sincere, and I could see she was so very glad it was all over.

On September 12, 2009, we called Yvonne and let her know we were going to be out in her area and asked if she would like to go to lunch. She said, "Sure," and we headed out that way. We went to lunch at a little restaurant just up the street from her house. Yvonne had a keen sense of people and she was very receptive to us and our emotions, so she knew something was up. Not to mention, she did tell me I should see a doctor early on in this journey. After we placed our order, I explained my diagnosis to her and tried diligently to reassure her I was going to be fine. She became emotional but kept it in check. Tears rolled down her face as she asked, "Are you going to be okay?"

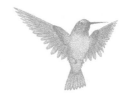

Chapter 6

Accepting Help

L ater in the day, my dear aunt Janie took me out to buy a notebook. She said it was important I keep track of what was going on and to journal, journal, journal. I had never been one to journal, but she was trying to help, and I knew I had to allow her that. Besides, she was so right.

I ended up picking out a pink transparent spiral bound notebook about composition size at the Staples down the street. Pink is not my favorite color or anything like that, but I gravitated to it. I was trying to find something inexpensive as my aunt was paying for it and I am not one to take advantage of someone's good nature. We then went to Michaels next door and picked out some stickers and ribbon to decorate it. I like angels, fairies, especially Tinkerbell, birds, mostly hummingbirds but

I find them all fascinating. I got some butterflies, Lorie was big on butterflies, and some sunflowers, Kaity's favorite flower, and Bears.

I know, after all the flying girlie things, then Bears. Well, my favorite football team is the Chicago Bears. I used to watch the games with my stepfather, Bob. He was from Detroit, Michigan, but loved his Bears and Cubs, which I had found very interesting. This was during the 1985 season. RJ was also born that year on Veterans day and the Bears went on to win the Superbowl to finish out the season. I also find bears to be magnificent animals with great strength, courage, and power, yet they appear to have a very sweet caring side to them. I also understand according to some Native American cultures that the bear is a sign of protection or courage.

The notebook was now decorated with Tinkerbell and butterflies. I had also created sections for journaling, orders, and results. I kept all of my disability paperwork in the notebook as well as created an area for research notes. My research was based on diet and how the heck did I get this disease and how was I going to avoid getting it again. As I thought of questions for the doctors, I jotted them down in the notebook also. There was a section of the notebook reserved for my Medical Fairies: General Practitioner Doctor, Surgeon, Radiologist, and Oncologist. The final section of the notebook was reserved for those who were my core center of Strength Fairies to call upon when I needed them. It was a short list, but those are the people I knew I could depend to be there for me and my family. Let me introduce you to my Strength Fairies.

Ric

The most loving, enduring, and supportive man a woman could be so fortunate to have in her life. He is not perfect, but that is what makes him perfect for me. Often times I wonder what I did so right to have him as my soul mate. By this time, we had known each other for more than 18 years. We are best friends and have suffered a lot of heartache the last couple of years, which only increased the bond between us. I had heard 70 percent of marriages break up when a child dies. I also heard a similar statistic when a woman has a life-threatening illness. In either case, and I can only speak for myself, but the option of splitting up never entered my mind. Ric never once gave me the inclination splitting up was an option for him either.

Through this whole ordeal he was by my side the entire time, never wavering. He went to all of the doctor appointments, lab draws, surgeries, radiation, and chemotherapy treatments with me. He was up front with his employer and co-workers, who were all very supportive and encouraging. It was never an issue for him to take time off to be with me. They encouraged him through this journey and for that we are very grateful.

Janie

Aunt Janie, as I mentioned before, had battled breast cancer only three years prior. She had basically appointed herself my mentor. That's Janie for you. She sees a need and she is there to take charge and try to make it all right. Not only are we related because she is my mom's sister, but we were now sisters in the world of breast cancer. My aunt and I have always had a special relationship. She is only 13 years older than me and when I was born, she had a say in what I was named. The Lynn of Bobbi Lynn was her idea. I remember hanging out with her as a kid in Ajo where we lived. There was a time when one of Janie's best friends, Johnny M., had taken Janie and I for a ride in his jeep over the arroyos in Ajo. We had so much fun; it was like being on a roller coaster. I will never forget that day. I remember Janie was always there for my mom, me, and my sisters and brother when we were growing up. She has a very giving heart, but don't piss her off. She had no problem taking on someone that crossed her. My cousin Susan swears to this day no one ever bothered her in school solely because she was Janie's cousin. She is one tough lady and a sheer force to be reckoned with if you overstep her boundaries. I don't recall ever being on the other end of that stick with her, but I had seen what she could do and wanted no part of it. Also, I believe I would have to have done something really unforgivably bad for her to rise against me.

Susan

My cousin Susan is nine years older than me. She is the daughter of my grandfather's younger brother, Mac. She used to babysit me when I lived in Ajo. I loved spending time with her as a child and always looked forward to the next time she would babysit me.

In the last 30-plus years we had only seen each other once or twice at family reunions, as our lives had gone different directions in that time. Unfortunately, in 2007, Mac at the age of 91 passed away from injuries sustained in a car accident. He was the last of that generation in our family. I would visit Mac from time to time. He even tried to teach me how to golf for a charity event I had signed up for (tried being the operative word as golf is one of the few things I struggle with). During our visits he raved about Susan and her family and I remembered hanging on every word. It was Mac being in the hospital after the car accident that brought Susan and I back together after so many years. The last time I visited Mac in the hospital before his passing, Susan and I had been at his bedside and were talking with him. He had a look of joy on his face and I believe it was from seeing Susan and I together again. After Mac's passing, Susan and I kept in touch and it was almost as if we picked up where we left off, not skipping a single beat. Yes, we had to get to know each other again, but the innate closeness we had was never lost. She is a wife, mother of two great cousins of mine, and grandmother of the two wonderful young men. She received her master's in counseling, which is so fitting for her. Susan also helped us get Kaity's Way off the ground, by arranging and paying for our first website and joining the board of directors.

She checked on me at least once a week and visited me when she was in the Phoenix area. She lived in my home town of Ajo, which is about two hours away. She was one of those people who loves to drive anywhere and everywhere. Just give her a reason and she was in the car and going. She put many miles on her vehicles. We are very opposite in that regard. If I had the money, I would actually pay someone to drive me around. I really just do not care for driving.

Mom

My mother, bless her heart, had only a few months earlier, lost a child (Lorie) after losing a granddaughter (Kaity). She was the executor of Lorie's estate, so she had been dealing with the insurance companies, Lorie's employer, and children. There was also the fact that at the time we had no clue what the reason was for Lorie's passing. We were in limbo with regards to the determination of her death, which eventually came back as undetermined. In the midst of all that, my mother was helping my youngest sister deal with her demons to quit the drug scene. Who had also become involved with drugs as a teenager and was going through withdrawals. My mother had become heavily involved in my sister's recovery as she decided she was not going to lose another child. We finally told my mother about my condition after the first attempt to remove the lump. She took the news as well as anyone would in her situation. I'm sure with losing Lorie and helping my younger sister out, my diagnosis was just another thing that had to be dealt with, and deal with it she would.

The Sunday after every one of my treatments, my mother would come over and cook a really nice dinner for my family. Ric really loved and appreciated it, as did I. Sunday dinners had been something we had done for years with our family, so her help with carrying it on while I was incapacitated was very thoughtful. Her presence would also allow Ric to run some errands or gave him some respite time. I enjoyed it because it felt as if, for the first time in my life, I had my mother's undivided attention and we would talk about anything and everything. If I asked, she would make me certain things to eat and freeze them for later. One time I had read the chemotherapy I was on would deplete my red blood cells and explained this to my mom. So, she went out and bought some liver and onions and cooked it up for me. I really liked her liver and onions. I could only eat a tiny bit, so she chopped up the rest and cooked some rice, added tomato sauce, and stuffed green bell peppers with the mixture then froze them for a later day. I really enjoyed this time with my mother. It had given us an opportunity to finally connect as mother and daughter, which was something I had longed for all my life.

Yvonne and Mooki

I mentioned them earlier. They are so alike in many ways that they struggle to this day with getting along. Yet, they are very different. Both of them are very strong-willed, but Mooki is very much a tomboy and Yvonne tends to be more in touch with her femininity. Mooki, being 16 years old, eventually came back to live with us— without TM (Yeah!)—while we were on this journey. She pitched in with caring for me when we needed her help. Yvonne, at 25 years old, lived in Surprise, a city about 20 miles west of where we live in Phoenix. Very much a free spirit and spiritually connected, was at that age where she was trying to find herself. She didn't have a solid mode of transportation but did what she could to come out to visit every couple of weeks. Truth be told, she struggled with me being ill but handled it the best way she knew how. Similar to how I felt about Janie being sick.

Angie

My sister-in-law, Angie (Ric's Sister), lives in Texas. No matter the distance, she did what she could to help. She was an ordained minister and prayed for us constantly. Ric and Angie are very close even though they have lived many miles from each other for most of their adult lives. You can see the sincere brother-sister love they have for each other. I was appreciative of Angie's support, especially for Ric. Because I had worked in home health care for 16 years, I knew that caregivers often times were overlooked. Not only did Ric have to care for me and drove me around to all my appointments and treatments, but he continued to work full-time, took care of the bills, house, kids' issues, and anything else that came our way. For Ric's sake, I was concerned, and it was such a relief that Angie was there for him, or so I thought. Later I figured out she was there for me also. Angie and I never really had an opportunity to connect since Ric and I had been together. Besides the distance, I was very guarded and was not an easy person to get to know. It was hard for me to let people in. I had a difficult time trusting people and I was suspicious of everyone and their motives—a very sad disposition—but not anymore.

Dodi

My shopping and wine-drinking buddy would call and check in on me at least every couple of weeks. She would always tell me, "If you need anything just call." Ric introduced me to Dodi. They worked together and he knew Dodi and I would be good friends. Working with Dodi and living with me, he could not catch a break and took it in stride. When Dodi and I first started hanging out, I did not like to shop for anything but groceries. Mostly, because I was afraid to spend money on anything but necessities, always fearing that we would need the money for something else. When it came to food, our cabinets, refrigerator, and freezer were stuffed. I had a real phobia of not having any enough food in the house. My idea of shopping for anything other than food was getting stuff for the kids or Ric. I did not like it when someone gave me money for a holiday, because I never spent it on myself. Well, Dodi taught me how to shop for myself. The first few times we went shopping, I probably spent no more than $20. Dodi on the other hand, would spend $100 or more. She would buy stuff she wanted, but she also shopped for her husband and son from time to time. I had a very practical attitude and knew how to do without. I had issues, no doubt. The thing about spending time with Dodi was I learned things about myself I never took the time to consider. Like what I wanted, and what I liked and that it was okay to pick myself up a little something. I learned about candles and how nice it was to burn them in your house to create an ambiance and pleasant scent. Oh, and let's not forget about the wine. When we first met, my wine experience consisted of Berringer's White Zinfandel and Sutter Homes Chenin Blanc. She exposed me to the reds, which I found absolutely fascinating. In early 2007, Dodi and I had planned and executed a trip to Napa Valley for later that year in the fall. We had so much fun. The icing on the cake was Dodi ran the liquor department where she worked and was able to get us several VIP tours of the various wineries. I found my favorite wine XYZin 50 by Geyser Peak. Dodi and I also got our first tattoos together. Hers hurt, so she said she would not be getting another. I have gotten two more since and have plans for two more. I guess you could say I am addicted.

Donna

The thought of her warms my heart and puts a smile on my face. She would come over from time to time to visit, bring food, or just check in on me. I have known Donna since 1998 I believe. We met because our children, her daughter Desi and RJ, went to school together. They were in junior high and Desi had a mad crush on RJ. RJ played Pop Warner football for the Savages and Desi was a cheerleader. Over time they became very good friends and were like brother and sister. They both watched out and cared very much for each other. Donna and her family loves RJ as much as we loves Desi. Desi and I had a very sweet relationship. She had become a niece of my heart. She was so hurt by my diagnosis that she was not able to come and see me until she knew I was going to be okay. And boy was she upset that we did not tell RJ. When she did finally come to see me, we both cried. I'm not sure what the emotion was, but I believe Desi also struggled with my diagnosis the same as I struggled with my aunt Janie's.

It is hard to explain, but Donna's family and my family just melded together over the years. I really do feel like we are all related. Donna saw me for the first time on the sidelines of one of RJ's football games. She was like, "Who is that woman?" I was easily excitable when it came to sports, especially games my kids played in. If RJ had the ball and was running down field, I was right there running down the sideline with him, encouraging him and cheering him on. Yes, I was that parent. Poor Yvonne, one time she had a basketball game and I would get so excited during the games that my cheering sometimes embarrassed her. After Donna found out I was RJ's mom, we met and became friends. For many years to Donna's family, before I got to know them all, I was known as RJ's Mom. To this day, sometimes when Donna introduces me to her friends or co-workers, she will tell them my name and then say, "RJ's mom." Then they knew who I was. I take great pride in the fact that Donna thinks so highly of RJ. Through the years, Donna has been by my side in good and bad times. She is that friend you may not talk with for a while, but when you do talk, it's like we always pick up where we left off. Donna is one of the few people who loved hanging out with me during RJ's football games. I say that because, I could clear the stands in front of us every time. I was very vocal in praising the team and encouraging them. Also, if the referees missed a call or penalty, they heard from me. We had to sit on the 50-yard line of every game at the top of the bleachers. For home games this put us just under the team video camera. I found this out after RJ came home one day and told me that as they were watching the game tape the following Monday, the coach asked, "Who is that person yelling all over the tape?" RJ, bless his heart, just took it in stride. Actually, I think the whole team found it comical and they just turned the volume down. We also attended all of the away games and often times Donna and her kids would ride with us or follow us to the games. We always had such a great time and reflect often on those times for a good laugh. We don't have high school football anymore to watch, but we still do things together. Donna is also a very dedicated volunteer for Kaity's Way and has gotten many of her family members and friends involved.

Kara

She, as I previously mentioned, took care of all of my benefits and disability paperwork. That was such a blessing and truly appreciated. Dealing with insurance companies is challenging on any level, but when you are dealing with a horrible illness it is great to have a Kara in your corner. After I returned to work from bereavement leave after losing Kaity, she gave me two necklaces that her and her mother made. Both of them had been made with hummingbird charms. One of them the string broke, but I wear the other to this day. I get so many compliments on my necklace and cherish the memory of Kara giving it to me.

Heidi

A dear friend I came to know on the job. She had become my boss and was duly warned about me as she had taken the position. She was told I was one of the supervisors she would be directing and would probably want to get rid of eventually. The funny thing is that she loved me. She realized I am not fake or phony and had little tolerance for office politics. Heidi helped me keep my job, of this I am sure, and I helped her in other ways as a friend. Heidi also came by from time to time to check on me. She also kept me in the know as to what was going on in the office. Upon my return to work, she lobbied to get me back on her team and took great care to work me in slowly. She understood the residual effects of chemotherapy.

Judy

A Reiki Master who came to know me through my aunt Janie. Judy sent me positive energy all the time. She is a very nice and caring lady.

Brandi

Then there is Brandi, my hair stylist. I had only started going to her about six months before my diagnosis, but we became fast and furious friends. She was another positive energy thrower and gave me a necklace with a pink quartz stone, which is said to be cleansing of negative energy. Every so often you are supposed to let it sit in salt to clear out the negative energy. It was funny how I came to know her. One day I was talking with my co-worker Stephanie about how I needed to find a hair stylist. She said she had a good friend from school that cut her hair. I liked the way Stephanie's hair was styled so I asked for the name of her stylist. The funny thing about this is the place Brandi worked at was called Curl Up and Dye. I had noticed it only a week before as I was on my way home from work. When I saw the name of the salon, I chuckled and thought it was a pretty creative play on words and name for a salon. Next thing I know I am getting my hair done there on a regular basis by Brandi.

Then there were the people who came on board after the fact, but in their own way just like the rest, helped me and my family as we weathered this journey.

Tammy

She is another one of my cousins and had battled cervical and ovarian cancer simultaneously just the year prior to my diagnosis. I am eight years older than Tammy, so the tables had turned. I babysat her when she was little. She is Janie's oldest child. So, after Janie dealt with her cancer, she was helping Tammy and her significant other the best she could. Tammy is a person with such a sweet disposition. She sent me a box filled with hats, books, trinkets, and a really cool hematite necklace. She lives in Colorado, so she called or texted me quite often to check on me. We had some really great conversations. It was as if we had gotten to know each other for the first time. I mean we knew each other as cousins, but we didn't know each other as people. By the time Tammy was a teenager, I had moved to California and spent 11 years there. When I moved back to Arizona, Tammy had moved to Colorado, so we kept missing each.

Cliff and Liz

My brother- and mother-in-law were there for us in their own way. Again, they were very supportive of Ric and extended a hand on more than one occasion.

Denise A.

Last, but certainly not least, there is Denise, my dearest friend from California. I have known Denise since 1989. She was not told of my condition until after the lump was removed. I didn't want to worry her. She has three beautiful daughters who are grown but she still had them to worry about as well as her mother who lived with her. Denise had called me one day in October to catch up. We had this knack for calling each other when we were on each other's mind. It was then that I told her what I had been going through. I remember when she called; Ric and I were at Goodwill, I do not recall what we were looking for. We found a book about babies for our daughter who was pregnant and a water bowl for the dogs. I was not a convincing liar so when she asked me how I was doing I told her about my diagnosis and the surgeries. Then I told her what was next. She was taken back and said she would be out to visit real soon. There was no doubt she would come.

In addition to everyone mentioned above, there were more family members, friends, and people I worked with who were absolutely wonderful and either came by to visit me when I was knee-deep in this journey or contacted me via text, email, or by phone to check on me from time to time. To name a few, Christy V., Lauren, Kathee, Denise W., Leslie, and Stephanie F. In one way or another, each of these people provided the support and encouragement someone in my position absolutely needed. I know there were many others who put me in their prayers, for which I am equally thankful.

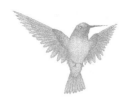

Chapter 7
On with the Journey

I was scheduled for a lumpectomy on September 17th. On September 14th I had a pre-lumpectomy appointment which I learned they were going to remove the lump and a sentinel lymph node. If that one is clear, they would remove one more lymph node just to be sure.

In the days leading up to that appointment, I realized I had all kinds of questions regarding the lumpectomy: Should I take Friday off? Where was Arrowhead Hospital? Did we need to bring the films? To avoid referral issues should we have communicated with our primary care physician (PCP)? Who was the anesthesiologist? The next two questions came from my aunt … Would I get a pillow for under my arm? Were they going to put a drainage tube in? I also wanted to be sure to show them the card that detailed an anesthesia cocktail given to me previously for a tubal ligation. That particular cocktail made me so very sick. It made me vomit a lot, yuck.

The doctor answered all of my questions. Yes, I needed to take Friday off. The hospital was located off 67th Avenue and Union Hills. Yes, we need to bring the films. Yes, we should keep my PCP in the loop. The doctor gave me the names of four different anesthesiologists, who I researched later and they checked out. No, I was not going to get a pillow for under my arm and a drainage tube placement depended on if they had to remove additional lymph nodes or not. Yes, if they had to, and no if not. One other thing we did on this day was a blood draw for the genetic testing, BRCA1 and BRCA2. If there was a mutation found in either of these genes, then this disease could be hereditary. I had also spoken with Becky at Arrowhead Hospital. She called to let me know $502 was due at the time of check-in and I needed to bring in my insurance card and identification. Later that evening at 7:00pm, Judy, the Rekik Master, sent me positive energy. I was not sure if it was mind over matter or the power of suggestion, but I did feel a warming sensation. Along with that, several people, including myself, prayed the tumor's growth would stop.

September 15th I had an appointment with the Radiologist off 83rd Avenue and Thunderbird. We were given our options of therapies and elected to do what is called brachytherapy, but we could only do it if the lymph nodes came back negative for cancer. From what I understood, this kind of therapy originated with the treatment of prostate cancer. Again, we had questions: Where were the therapies done? *At the same office were are at.* When was the balloon for the radiation going to be inserted? *One week after surgery.* What were the side effects of this kind of therapy? *None other than fatigue.* That's sweet. How soon would radiation start after the balloon was inserted? *One day.* What came first: radiation or hormone treatment? *We won't know the answer to that until after surgery.* Would I have to pay a co-pay for each treatment? *Maybe not, they would have to look into it.* I was given a prescription for ten days' worth of Keflex. A strong antibiotic to take over the course of radiation to make sure I didn't get an infection. There were also three appointments made for me after the surgery to get started with radiation. September 22nd at 11:00am, ultrasound with the radiation oncologist. September 23rd at 7:00am, balloon inserted by the surgeon, the same day at 1:30pm I was scheduled for a CT scan with the radiation oncologist. I was also scheduled to see the oncologist on October 6th. I received a call from Mary Helen at Arrowhead Hospital to pre-register for surgery. She also told me I needed to get a chest x-ray, blood drawn, and drop a UA (give a urine sample). Off to Arrowhead Hospital we went.

Okay, so I believed I was all ready for surgery. I was so hoping they did not find the cancer had gotten to the lymph nodes. If cancer was not found in the lymph nodes, then we only had two weeks of radiation therapy as opposed to seven weeks. The other reason being if cancer was found in the lymph nodes, they would have had to remove the whole tree of them. Cancer in the lymph nodes was also indicative of cancer traveling through the bloodstream. At least that was the way I understood things to be. The removal of the whole tree of lymph nodes also opened me up for possible additional problems in the future. Nonetheless, I was not willing to discuss the later unless it became necessary. We would know which direction we were going after surgery on the seventeenth. Judy was sending me more positive energy. She also said I should say over and over again "I am cancer free!" all day long every day. She also suggested I ask angels to help me rid myself of all negative thoughts or energy. She advised me to cut white products out of my diet: flour, bread, sugar, rice, or pasta. They are over-processed and don't help with healing.

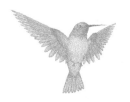

Chapter 8

Lump o what a Me?

There we were the day of surgery, September 17th. "I am cancer free!" I said to start my day. The lump was to be removed and lymph nodes tested. We were hoping the lymph nodes tested negative for cancerous cells. We checked in at 9:30am sharp. Prior to checking in, I had gotten a call from Janie and Judy, both were very concerned about me having negative energy. Judy mentioned possibly picking up on my fear. I am sure she was, because I had never been so scared in my life. Everything was moving so fast and I felt terrified when the biopsy had come back cancerous. I was almost afraid to hope for a positive outcome from this surgery, but I still tried to remain positive.

"I am cancer free!" I said again and again.

After I checked in, we waited for a bit and at 10:30am, Dave from nuclear medicine called me back to do a nuclear dye injection to locate the correct lymph nodes to test. Dave was very nice. He told us about being a nuclear medical technician and talked about his three children. He had a 22-year-old daughter who graduated from ASU with a business degree, his son was 19 years old and attended ASU to get a degree in chemical engineering. He also had a 14-year-old daughter who lived with her mother in West Virginia. As I laid there watching the dye make its way to my lymph nodes, something inside kept telling me to talk about Kaity's Way and the fund-raising raffle we were having. I did just that and after a few moments of silence I asked Ric to give Dave a Kaity's Way brochure. After he read it, he shared with us that his youngest daughter had a boyfriend who was in jail for violence and asked us for a second brochure to send to his daughter. He said he had told her she cannot fix him. I shared with him an idea I share with any parent who felt there may be an issue of teen dating violence going on with their child. I suggested he bring up our website (www. kaitysway.org) on his computer. We had constructed it in such a way to be attractive to both male and female. The home page had a short summary of what happened to Kaity. Now once he brought it up, just let it sit there until she sat at the computer and was faced with Kaity's story. Hopefully she would take to reading the story, giving the him a perfect opportunity to strike up conversation about teen dating violence with her. I believed he put this idea to memory. Then he bought six raffle tickets. I can remember hoping he won something in the raffle. Bless both of their hearts, I sincerely hoped the brochure and website helped the young lady realize her father was right. After we finished up with Dave, I wished I had asked his daughter's name so I could have said a prayer specifically for her. I said a prayer for them anyways.

I was taken back and prepped for surgery. The nurses were really nice and compassionate. They had to call a certain nurse in to start my IV because for some reason my veins were not cooperating. I was in a curtained-off area and Ric was brought back. We were reading, doing puzzles and talking from time to time to make light of the situation—all this in between the nurses getting me ready for surgery. Then we received a phone call from TM, that so-called friend of Mooki's. She felt compelled to let us know Mooki had just done a home pregnancy test and the result was positive. I really believed she was overjoyed to deliver such news to us. She was a manipulative person who took advantage of Mooki's vulnerable state and now she was throwing it in our faces that Mooki was pregnant. Ric was very nonchalant about it and said, "Okay." He is so great at not giving people like TM what they want. Not to mention, at the moment, we had much bigger fish to fry unbeknownst to Mooki and TM. I don't know if it was the moment we were in or what, but we did not react to the news TM gave us. We just figured everything happens for a reason and until we talk with Mooki, we were not going to allow it to sway our focus at the moment. Janie and my mother arrived, and again there was more small talk and cracking jokes. At approximately 12:25pm the surgeon stopped in and explained they were running about an hour behind schedule and after the surgery they would put a special wrap type of bra on me. I was instructed not to take it off for two days, which also meant I could not shower for two days. Janie asked the surgeon about the drainage tube. The surgeon explained that if they had to take all of the lymph nodes because they found traces of cancer in the first two, then yes there would be a drainage tube placed. So, the hope was when I come out of surgery, there was no drainage tube. The surgeon also explained when we meet the following Wednesday, she would insert the balloon for the brachytherapy at her Arrowhead office. She said I should be sure to take a painkiller before that appointment. The surgeon left and I realize we did not get the suite number to her Arrowhead office. We made a note of that.

The anesthesiologist stopped by to talk with me and explained the procedure and asked if I had any questions. I showed her the card I kept of the cocktail given to me during a previous surgery which made me very sick. I also mentioned I had woken up during surgery one time in the past. She took note of this information and assured me she would mix me a better cocktail. The four of us made small talk until it was time. We also found out the suite number; it is 101.

It was time. I kissed my husband and we said I love you. I hugged my mom and Janie. I became emotional, because the looks on their faces were hopeful but trimmed with fear. My mother was telling me I was going to be fine as if I were five years old. This made me even more emotional, because it was not often that my mother showed this kind of emotion toward me. We arrived at the operating room and I was shifted to another bed and I remembered the room being very bright. It seemed like there were lights everywhere. They hooked me up to the monitoring machines, put an oxygen mask on me, then the cocktail was started, and I was out.

The next thing I remembered was being very groggy and trying to talk but I could not find my voice. The recovery nurse checked on me and saw I was coming to. All of a sudden, Ric, Mom, Janie and Yvonne were at my bedside and they all look so relieved. I was happy to see Yvonne there. She looked relieved, but I could see the fear in her eyes. Ric had gone to pick Yvonne up while I was in surgery. When I finally found my voice, my first question was, "is there a drainage tube?" Janie, with a look of sheer delight, said, "no." This was great news and I was elated. This was the first bit of good news we had gotten since the diagnosis. My family's relief wasn't so much the lack of a drainage tube, but apparently I had been very slow to come out of the anesthesia. I guess that was one heck of a cocktail the anesthesiologist gave me because it took an hour longer than they anticipated for me to come to. Who knows, maybe I just needed some rest. Lord knows I had not been sleeping very well since the diagnosis. Once I was able, Ric helped me get dressed and we were out of there and I was starving. I hadn't eaten since midnight and it was nearly 2:00 in the afternoon.

While I was still recovering the next day in bed, Yvonne came over to hang out with me. Eventually, she fell asleep and Ric, the sweet soul he is, slept in the guest room for the night. I was still stoked about the fact that there is no drainage tube. The lymph nodes were negative: no cancer. The lump was gone, or so I thought.

Judy, bless her heart, cried tears of joy when Janie relayed the good news to her about no cancer found in the lymph nodes. I could only imagine how exhausted she was, with all the positive energy she was sending me. "I am cancer free!" This was a new beginning. All I had to do was five days of brachytherapy as a precautionary measure. Whoop, whoop! Things were looking good. I had vowed to take better care of myself; I would exercise more by putting yoga back into my routine. This would help to alleviate stress as I felt stress is what brought this on. I was going to work really hard to not stress about anything. Life is too precious and short to hold grudges. I took my pain medicine and chilled.

Later that day, I received a call from a woman with the oncology case management department team of my medical insurance company. She explained to me she was available to answer questions about procedures and benefits. I didn't have any questions at the moment, I was on painkillers, so it was no wonder. She gave me her phone number just in case.

"I am cancer free!"

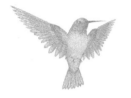

Chapter 9
Ah ... Yeah ... No

It was September 22nd and I was scheduled to see the radia-tion oncologist today. He said the pathology report confirmed there was no cancer found in the lymph nodes but... it appeared the surgeon did not get the entire tumor. What the heck? What does that mean? "Two of the four margins, new deep margin and new lateral margin, around the lump excised showed cancer cells." This was a setback. They were going to have to go back in and take more tissue from these two areas before they could place the balloon. The new deep margin was closest to the chest wall. The new lateral margin was closest to my arm. They contacted the surgeon's office to inform them of the results and the change in plans. I was told the surgeon's office would call me with a date for the next surgery. I was so glad Ric was with me. That kind of news was not easy to take. I could not even imagine being alone and receiving this kind of news. On the flip side, I felt bad for Ric as he was just as disappointed as I was. All in all, we focused our thoughts on the fact that the lymph nodes still tested negative for cancer.

By 4:00 in the afternoon, I still had not received a call from the surgeon's office. So, I called and left a message with the person in charge of scheduling. About an hour later I received a call from the radiation oncologist office. They told me I should go in for my scheduled appointment with the surgeon since they hadn't called me yet.

Later in the evening, I realized a few questions for the medical insurance case manager and had to leave her a message to call back. My questions were: Did we have to pay another $500 for surgery? And with the possibility the cancerous cells still remaining, would they have to take more lymph nodes?

We were at the surgeon's office bright and early at 7:00 in the morning. The receptionist was confused, because the surgeon's office was under the impression the radiation oncologist's office was going to talk with me more, about what, I was not sure. In any event, the next surgery was scheduled for September 30th at noon.

The surgeon mentioned I should ask the oncologist about a port to administer the drugs. She also said I need to ask about the onco type. I didn't have a clue what she was talking about. Onco type, port, drugs, what drugs, chemotherapy, or hormone therapy? I could only have hormone therapy if the results showed my estrogen receptors (ERP) were positive. She said we will need to find out from the oncologist if a port should be placed. Okay, well I guess this meant I needed to get in to see the oncologist sooner rather than later. I called the oncology office and they set an appointment for September 29th at 3:30 in the afternoon.

Later that day I received a couple of phone calls. The first one was from the radiation oncologist's office and they told me the ERP came back positive, which made me a good candidate for hormone therapy. This was good, or so I thought. Then I received a call from Arrowhead Hospital regarding the surgery. They said I will need to pay $394.56 for the next surgery and that should take care of my max out of pocket, which was good because everything after that would be paid at 100 percent.

Since finding the lump, I feel as if we had been on an emotional roller coaster. For a while we were coasting low, and then we got a bit of good news that took us up to the top, only to turn 90 degrees straight down for another scary ride. With the ERP coming back positive, we felt like we were at the top. We were hoping the oncologist visit will allow us to stay up, but I learned to remain cautiously optimistic.

The other call was the Case Manager returning my call. Her answers to my questions were that we would have to wait until we see the oncologist on the 29th to get answers. She also told me she would be out of the office until next Tuesday. I did get a bit of good news though, the insurance company approved the brachytherapy after all. I hadn't even known it was an issue.

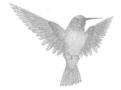

Chapter 10

And the Beat Goes On

O h wow, with all of this going on, I completely forgot the Arizona Coalition Against Domestic Violence (AZCADV) was trying to set up a press conference in regard to Kaity's Law, which was to be signed any day by the governor. Kaity's Law is a law that the AZCADV asked me to testify on behalf of, so those in abusive dating relationships would have the same protection under the law as those abused in domestic relationships. Sadly, it took the loss of Kaity's life to get this bill passed. I contacted AZCADV and informed them of what was going on with me and asked if they could postpone the press conference if they felt it was important that I be there. They were not sure this was possible because of everyone's schedule. I understood and left it at that. As it turned out, they were not able to coordinate a press conference due to scheduling conflicts. The governor eventually signed the bill on September 30th, the same date of my next surgery.

Remember the paperwork Kara took care of for me regarding my disability? Well, I received a call from the disability carrier on September 24th informing me that they received the paperwork and it was in process. They also gave me my claim number and a contact number if I had any questions. This was also the same day I received a phone call from my dear friend Denise. I really thought I would have gotten through this before her and I saw each other again, so I wasn't going to tell her. Although, when I heard her voice, I had to tell her. Denise and I had known each other for 20 years. There was no use in me trying to lie to her, because she would see right through me. The other reason I considered not telling Denise was because it was so hard telling the people you love and who love you that you were battling cancer. They were so saddened by the news and their first thought seemed to be that you had been handed a death sentence. After talking with Denise, I realized today was the first day since surgery I felt halfway decent. My underarm where they took the lymph nodes still hurt a little. I could tell the nerves were reconnecting at the incision, just in time for my next surgery.

September 25th was a quiet day. There was not much going on and I heard from only one person today, Lauren. She is such a sweet person. We really love her like she was our own child. I actually worked on Kaity's Way stuff to keep my mind off the cancer. I worked on a banner and I scheduled a presentation for October 3rd for the Governor's Youth Commission. I prepared my speech and organized all the literature we were going to distribute to them. My cousin Susan and Ric would go with me to the presentation. When I was all done, I grabbed a beer and sat down to watch Sideways. I really like that movie. I should probably have had a glass of wine instead.

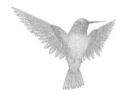

Chapter 11

Is it Genetic?

I received a call from the surgeon's office on September 28th. The genetic test results had come back negative. There were no noticeable mutations. Yippee! I was so glad because this was good news for my daughters. It also narrowed down the playing field for how I got this disease. I also received a call from Arrowhead Hospital. They told me I had to go in for a chest x-ray for pre-op and confirmed my surgery on the 30th. I called Yvonne to give her the good news and asked her to come over on the 29th to stay up with me until 3:00am since the surgery was scheduled for later in the day on the 30th. She said she would be over.

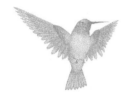

Chapter 12

Other Matters
of the Heart

L
ater in the evening, Mooki and her boyfriend had come over to have dinner with us. We had spaghetti, salad, and corn. Without disappointment or judgment, we discussed their options given the results of the home pregnancy test she had taken. She was adamant about keeping the baby and we supported her decision. We then discussed with them the commitment they were making and since a baby was on the way, their wants and needs were secondary to the baby's. This meant the partying needed to stop. For every decision they made from here on out, the first question that should come into their minds was, what is best for the baby from now until the child becomes an adult and is able to take care of his or herself. We discussed Mooki's plans to see a doctor, who she had already decided on. It was the same doctor

TM was seeing. Yes, TM was about three months more pregnant than Mooki. Yeah, I suspected a set-up too but what can you say? What was done was done. No need to dwell on something we had no control over. Eventually, we talked with Mooki about her and her boyfriend moving in with us. We mentioned this because we felt living in our household was the best opportunity for the baby. We kept good food in the house and our environment was to be kept as stress-free as possible, given what we were going through. We could also make sure she gets to her doctor appointments and needless to say, we love Mooki and only wanted the best for her and our first grandchild. She was not so sure about coming back to live with us, because her and TM had this grand idea that they were going to raise their babies together. Through the conversation, it became apparent they were trying to wedge the baby's daddy out of the picture. Mooki and TM were going to be the parents of these unborn babies! I could see in the young man's demeanor he felt defeated by these two. At the time, I just took in what Mooki said and let it go for another time.

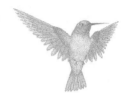

Chapter 13

What to Do?

Since surgery was not scheduled until noon, I could eat up until 3:00 in the morning. Yvonne was coming over to stay up with me. This way I could have my final meal just before 3:00 in the morning and hopefully I would sleep in until 10:30 or 11:00. Then I could get up, get ready, and go to the hospital. I didn't want to sit around smelling food or be thirsty for several hours before surgery.

As we were waiting to see and meet the oncologist, I noticed a plaque on the wall, in the year 2000 he was voted by his peers as one of Phoenix's Best Doctors. This was encouraging. They called us back and took my vitals. My weight was 154.5, blood pressure 120/82 and pulse was 64. So far so good, besides my weight being a little high for my height (5'3"), my numbers were looking pretty good. After the nurse was done with me, she stepped out, and we waited for the doctor to come in. We met the oncologist for the first time. He was a better-than-average-looking man, slender, average height. I guessed he was in his mid to late fifties. He had a full head of fine hair that was in a ponytail at least half way down his back. I heard he raised horses, which was cool because that meant we had something in common. He was a quiet man with a very somber personality. I could see how that would be given his profession and line of study. My first impression was I am fine with him. I did not get any bristling feelings about him or in his presence. I was learning to listen to my gut, especially after losing Kaity.

Just when I thought things were looking up, the oncologist told us chemotherapy was necessary, mostly due to the size of the tumor. He explained that even though the lymph nodes showed negative, there was a chance cells were roaming around my body. He explained, when cancer returned, it usually came back elsewhere and then it was usually fatal and quality of life was poopy—my word, not his.

I did have the option to skip the chemotherapy and just do hormone therapy, but that would have meant an increased chance of the cancer returning; whereas, if I went the chemotherapy route, it should kill the floaters. The look on Ric's face was guarded. I am pretty sure I knew what he is thinking.

You see, for years when we had discussed someone being diagnosed with cancer, I had said, "If I am ever diagnosed with cancer, just buy me a bag of weed and let me be." I had this attitude because I spent three years of my life as a pharmaceutical technician and the last 16 years working in the home healthcare arena. I heard the horror stories and some of the chemotherapy medications literally had to be handled with gloves because they are that poisonous. I had often heard the treatment was worse than the disease. I was so on the fence at this point. Should I stick to my guns and just let the cancer take over and die or do I suck it up and do the treatment?

I looked at Ric and asked him his opinion. I was so sorry I did that. It was very selfish of me to put him in that position. I was desperate. All I could think of was my family, him, and the kids. I wanted to be here for them. Ric said to do chemotherapy. I then looked at the oncologist and asked him if he were in my shoes what would he do? Without hesitation he said he would do it. I was leaning towards chemotherapy but wanted some sort of sign it was the right direction to go. Since it was unanimous, I opted to do it. I also figured it was better to go through it at the age of 45, instead of trying to tackle it when I was older. Let's just get it over with and get rid of these cells that could cause havoc later. The oncologist knew I was having surgery the very next day, so we set the target date to start chemotherapy for October 20th. This allowed time for me to heal from surgery and then do the radiation.

On the second surgery day, September 30th, Yvonne and I successfully stayed up until 3:00am. It was nice to spend the evening with her. We watched TV and talked. It was quality time and I enjoyed every minute of it. I love spending time with my kids, and it's really nice when the time is one-on-one. I must have been nervous about the surgery because my plan did not work. I was up at 8:30am. So, I did some stuff with Kaity's Way; answered emails, researched some issues, and looked to see if the governor had signed the bill for Kaity's Law (nothing yet), which was signed by the governor later that day. Dodi called and left a message at 10:02am. I called her back on the way to the hospital. She was in New York visiting family and just wanted to see how I was doing. I told her it was all good and gave her the recent updates. By this time, I was bored with what was going on and just wanted to get it over with. My hope was we could move into the next phase after this surgery, which would be radiation.

We arrived at the hospital and basically the routine was the same. I was taken back to the prepping area. I got in the hospital attire and into bed, an IV was placed, we went over the same questions, and then Ric was brought back to be with me while we waited. It was just Ric and I this time. Mom was up north, and Janie had to work, Yvonne was trying to get a ride to the hospital, but things didn't pan out. It was all good. The surgeon stopped in to say hi. Then the anesthesiologist stopped in and talked about the cocktail given to me during the last surgery. While it did not make me sick, it kept me under for quite a while. So, this time they would back off on a couple of the drugs so that I could come out of it sooner.

It was time. Ric and I kissed, exchanged I love you's and I was wheeled into the operating room again. I was shifted to another bed, the cocktail was served, and I was out. I was not in surgery long and I came out of the anesthesia faster. We were out of there by 4:00pm and again I was starving. At nearly 5:00pm, the Radiation Oncology doctor's office called and I was told the brachytherapy balloon was scheduled for placement on October 14th bright and early at 7:00am. I would then get a cat scan later that day at 1:50pm. On October 13th the Radiation Oncology doctor wanted to see me at 10:00am for an ultrasound.

By this time, things had become very overwhelming. There were all the doctor appointments and then there was some confusion as to when the balloon was to be placed which eventually got worked out. Then for some reason I noted I needed to call the oncologist doctor to move the chemotherapy up to start the 15th of October. Oh, and there was a note about a PET scan and heart test. Then I needed to call the dentist to discuss the care of my teeth and gums while going through treatment. Man, oh man, I felt like I was going to lose my mind and I had a support system. Every time I started feeling overwhelmed, I told myself to just chill, it would all work out.

On October 1st I talked with the surgeon's office and was told the balloon was scheduled to be placed on October 7th at 7:00am instead at the Arrowhead office. I left a message for the Radiation Oncology doctor's office with this information. I also needed to go in for a MUGA scan on October 6th at 10:30am at Arrowhead Hospital. The Radiation Oncology doctor's office called me back and told me I needed to be in to see them at 2:00pm on October 6th to go over the pathology results and have an ultrasound done. I would see them again on October 7th for a CAT scan at 1:50pm.

Goodness gracious, would it ever end? Yes, it would, but not soon enough for me. We were literally bouncing all over the place. Through it all, Ric was with me every step of the way. That was why it was so important to us that his employer was very empathetic and supportive. I have to give a shout out to Ric's co-workers. I knew they were good people, because when we lost Kaity they rallied around us and did whatever they could to make our lives tolerable. They saw our house was filled with family and friends, so they arranged for a refrigerator to be brought to the house, along with extra bedding, a canopy for the front yard, and the food was overwhelming, hence the refrigerator. Then a few of them came by on their own time to offer their support and talked with us. Now, with my diagnosis, they once again kicked it into gear and would send words of encouragement home with Ric, not to mention how they covered for him at work so he could be with me as much as I needed him. All the while I was also receiving numerous calls and text messages of encouragement from family and friends.

It was October 2nd and I was still on painkillers from surgery a couple of days ago and was trying to prepare for the speaking engagement at the Governors Youth Commission the next day. I was so glad Ric and Susan were both going to be there to help with the presentation. Oh, and it was my 46th birthday. Given the circumstances, it was hard to be joyful about it. Nonetheless, Yvonne came over to join Ric, Mooki, and I for my birthday. RJ called to wish me a Happy Birthday and as I was talking to him I felt apprehensive about keeping my situation a secret. I just kept telling myself that it was for his own good. Dan was still angry with us, so I did not hear from him. My mother came over to the house and so did my Aunt Janie and Susan. It turned out to be a nice and fun evening. Actually, for a brief moment, I forgot about what had been dominating our lives and that felt nice. I got a couple of cool gifts too. Ric gave me a top-of-the-line Pittsburgh Steelers Polamalu Jersey, the kind that has the lettering stitched on the back. I like it a lot. The Steelers are my second favorite team and next to Brian Urlacher from the Chicago Bears, I really like to watch Troy Polamalu play football. He was a phenomenal athlete and appeared to be very gracious and humble, which was not an easy thing to pull off when you played football as well as he did.

It was time to share Kaity's Story with the Governors Youth Commission. Since I had surgery only three days prior and was still on painkillers, I was not on top of my game. I was also trying really hard to hide the bandages and not move too quickly. Yet I didn't want to appear like I was feeble. There were a couple of areas I stumbled on my words and I completely forgot the Power Point presentation. Even so, the surveys came back favorable. The kids really got the message we were trying to convey and that was all that mattered. It really helped having Ric and Susan there. Not only did they help with the handouts, but the moral support was immense. I really just needed them there. I think they were both concerned about me and wanted to be there just in case I fell out or something. I was being stubborn as the show must go on. I also did not say anything to the leader of the Governors Youth Commission about my condition. How do you tell someone you don't know very well you have cancer? "Oh, by the way, I have cancer and had a second surgery only a few days ago." It just does not seem to flow off the tongue too well. Not to mention, if it were me in her shoes, I would have given me an out or cancelled the engagement and that was the last thing I wanted. Breast cancer was not going to get in the way of our mission; no way, no how, absolutely not.

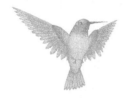

Chapter 14

Prep Time

O ver the next couple of days, I started doing some research about diet and what I needed to do to get through this as smoothly as possible. What a laugh; smooth is just not a word within the chemotherapy arena. Okay maybe when it comes to your bald head, but otherwise smooth just does not happen. Nonetheless, I made a couple of lists with regard to items I need to work into my diet weekly and daily. This is information I pulled off the internet from watching Dr. Oz (love him) as well as information I received from other cancer survivors and friends and family.

WEEKLY	DAILY
Avocado	Asparagus, four tbsp twice daily
Broccoli	Water, eight to 10 eight oz glasses a day
Kale	Green tea, two cups per day hot or cold
Leeks	Cinnamon
Brussel Sprouts	Honey
Cauliflower	Lysine 1 tablet daily
Collard Greens	Glutamine
Cabbage	100 percent Fruit Juice
Salmon	
Swordfish	
Flaxseed	
Organic Chicken	

Armed with this information I made a check list:_

<u>Nutritional Daily Check List</u>

Date:

- Cinnamon and Honey Tea 1st ½
  - o 1 part Cinnamon 2 parts Honey
  - o Directions: Pour 6 oz. boiling water over 1 tsp Cinnamon stir, let cool. Once cooled add 2 tsp honey and stir
- 1 oz Aloe Vera Juice AM
- 1 oz Aloe Vera Juice Midday
- 1 oz Aloe Vera Juice PM
- Vitamins and Lysine
- 10gm Glutamine AM

- 10gm Glutamine Midday
- 10gm Glutamine PM
- 4 tbsp asparagus AM (straight or in juice)
- 4 tbsp asparagus PM (straight or in juice)
- Bottle of Water
- Bottle of Water
- Bottle of Water
- Bottle of Water
- 2 cups or Glasses of Green Tea
- 1 Fruit Smoothie
- 1 serving of Broccoli or Leek or Cauliflower or Collard Greens or Brussel Sprouts or Cabbage or Kale
- 1 serving of Chicken or Salmon or Sword fish or turkey
- Cinnamon and Honey Tea 2nd ½

Next, I looked into what needed to be done to lessen the instances of side effects from the chemotherapy. Someone suggested that two hours before treatment I should eat a meal with protein and bread. Avoid fat, grease, and sugar. Some ideas I listed were: a chicken dish with bread, salmon salad with bread, a turkey sandwich, salad with bread, yogurt with nuts, and lentil soup.

How should I dress for the treatments? Sweat pants, a shirt which allows access to the port, and comfortable shoes or, better yet, slippers should do it. I would also want to bring a book, blanket, puzzle book, snacks, and popsicles (to minimize mouth blisters).

Next, I decided after each treatment I wanted to do something to treat myself. That was of course if my blood count was in the good range. A pedicure and/or manicure, maybe a facial, or I recently heard the American Cancer Society provided free makeovers. I would call to check into that.

Then I was told I should consider keeping the following items on hand:

ITEM	REASON
Baking soda	1-2 tsp dissolved in water swished around in mouth lessens mouth sores
Mints/Gum/Lemon Drops	To help the metallic taste in mouth from therapy
Slippery Elm	For sore throat due to therapy
Mineral Oil/Lotion (Body, Face, Hand)	For moisturizing skin
Sunscreen w/UVA and UVB protection	To protect skin from burning when out in the sun
Mint Tea	Settle the stomach
Mint flavored milk of magnesia	Constipation
Animal Crackers	Bland enough to eat after treatment
Ginger Ale or Ginger tea	Settle Stomach
Aloe Vera Juice	Good for digestion
Coconut Water	Hydration
Bananas/Apples/Potatoes/Peas	Provides fluid and nutrients
Watermelon/Pineapple/Kiwi/ Prunes/Apricots/Nuts	Provides fiber to lessen constipation
Produce cleaner	Clean Produce

October 6th and were once again back at Arrowhead Hospital for the MUGA scan. This is a test to see how well my heart pumps blood. One of the chemotherapy drugs (Adriamycin) was so toxic that it could cause heart damage. If the heart was compromised, then we'd have issues. It made me happy to see that Dave, the nuclear medicine technician, was doing this scan also. We struck up conversation and he told me he was headed to New York for the weekend with his wife; otherwise, this would have been his day off. I wondered if he would be the one doing the test, but dismissed it thinking it might have been his day off. Was I right on or what? I don't know how, but it was weird that I thought in so much detail. I was not sure what to think, but Dave was a nice guy and I was glad he was taking care of me again. He took me to the same room as before and took a big tube of blood then a small syringe of blood. He explained they were going to mix my blood with a nuclear dye then inject it back into me and watch it go through my heart to see how well my heart pumped it out. As Dave was doing the blood mixing, I thought how nice it was nice to see a friendly face in the midst of all we were going through. He came back and the nuclear enriched blood was injected. As we were going through the motions Dave told me he sent the Kaity's Way brochure to his ex-wife in Virginia to share with their daughter. He was happy to report the abusive guy had gone to prison and his daughter has moved on. Now there was a blessing for you, thank God. I love hearing good things like that. I was not sure Kaity's Way had anything to do with it, but that was not the point. The point was that the victim got away from the abuser.

Okay, that was a two-hour process and Dave mentioned we may have to do this again in six months. He also said the

Oncologist should get the report the following day. Next, we had an appointment with the Radiation Oncology doctor's office at 2:00pm. After we had a quick bite to eat, we were at the Radiation Oncology doctor's office. Unfortunately, the news was not all good. The good news first, the new deep margin area (chest wall) was clear of cancerous cells. The not-so-good news, the new lateral margin area (closest to my arm) still showed some cancerous cells. Apparently, the tissue they took from the last surgery was not enough for the lateral margin. According to the x-ray, there was what I call a runner. It looked like the lump had a tail extending towards my arm or worse the lymph nodes. The Radiation Oncology doctor said it was up to the surgeon as to what we were going to do. Are we going to have another surgery? If so, would it be a matter of taking more tissue or doing a mastectomy? Oh well, it was what it was, no sense in getting upset at anyone. Ric was frustrated. He could not understand why this kept happening. I believe everything had finally come to the surface for him and he just needed to vent. I let him get it off his chest and it was all good.

I decided to start a blog today, a digital journal so to speak. I named it "C is for Conquer." I kept it private and as anonymous as I could, just in case one of the boys happened upon it, they would not be able to tie it to me. I came to this decision because there were constant updates and people wanted to be kept in the know. Creating a blog was the perfect tool for the job. It allowed me to keep journaling in such a way that others could stay current at their leisure. For example, my friend Dodi's work schedule required her to be up anytime between midnight and 2:00am to get ready. At times, she would get on the computer before work to check emails and the like. The blog would allow her to check in on me at this time also. People still wanted to hear from me directly but that was okay because the conversations weren't dominated by my condition. I was tired of talking about myself. I liked to hear what was going on in their lives more.

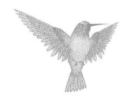

Chapter 15

And a Blogging
We Will Go

TUESDAY, OCTOBER 6, 2009

Where are we now?

I have created this blog in an effort to keep all those concerned, about my condition, informed. I get emails and texts and calls daily which I Sincerely Appreciate. Honestly, because so much is going on, I cannot remember who I talked to in one way or another or not. The last thing I want to do is think I responded to someone and didn't. There is another therapeutic reason for doing this. It gives me the opportunity to put in writing what is going on and helps me work through this trying time in my life.

Here is the latest—I had to get a MUGA Scan today. New to me so I will explain it. They drew some blood from me, a small syringe full, and mixed it with some nuclear radioactive stuff. One component is #99 on the periodic table. I haven't looked it up yet. Anyways, then they inject the radioactive blood back into me, to see how my heart pumps it through my system. This is necessary because one of the chemo drugs they want to give me can be hard on the heart. It was about a 2 hr process and the Tech said it will probably need to be done again in 6 mos. This is the same Nuclear Tech that injected the radioactive dye for finding the lymph nodes, he is a nice guy.

That was the first part of the day ... The second part of the day I had to see the Radiation Oncologist (RO) to find out if the 2nd surgery was successful in getting the rest of the tumor. The deep margin (chest wall) showed no abnormal cells the lateral margin on the other hand did show some abnormal cells, bummer. The RO doctor also did an ultrasound on the cavity to check for placement of the balloon for the Brachytherapy.

TomorrowI have an appt with the Surgeon and she will let me know if we need to have a 3rd surgery or if we are going to let the Radiation eradicate to abnormal cells. So we shall see.

For those of you that are just getting this info I will provide a little background info. In mid August I discovered a lump in my breast and went to the family Dr. who confirmed yes there is a lump there. She promptly sent me for a mammogram and ultrasound and referred me to a Surgeon who did a biopsy on Sept 8th, and on Sept 11th she told us the lump was invasive ductal carcinoma and obviously it has an attitude (the attitude part is me not the Dr.).

Moving on, on Sept 17th I had surgery #1, which they got most of the tumor but 2 margins, deep tissue and lateral, showed abnormal cells in the margins. They also took 2 sentinel lymph nodes which were clear (Yippee!). This brings us to surgery #2 which they got it all in the deep tissue margin, but not the lateral margin.

When we first started this Journey, we were of the mind it was a matter of removing the lump making sure the lymph nodes were clear, 5 days of Radiation and we are done. Well, there have been further developments and the Oncologist strongly suggests I go through chemotherapy as a systemic precaution as abnormal cells do not just travel through the lymph nodes it can also travel through the blood. If these abnormal cells are given the opportunity to rear their ugly heads again, it is usually in the bones, brain or necessary organs, not good. So needless to say I elected to do the chemotherapy, as scary as that might be.

I know I will get through this as I have the True and Unconditional Love of my Family and Friends. My husband is with me all the way and I am so blessed to have him in my life forever and ever. My Aunt and Cousin have both had similar battles and have been there for me since I finally had the courage to tell them. Everything they learned from what they experienced they are passing on to me and I appreciate them so much for being there. My mother, mother-in-law, sister-in-law and brother-in-law have been very Helpful and Supportive as well… It is not easy for them as they all live quite a ways away from us, but that doesn't stop them. Then there are my dear dear friends who have all asked what can I do. Well, you are doing it by keeping me in your prayers, sending me positive thoughts and energy and checking in on me from time to time. The outpouring of Love I feel from everyone is positively overwhelming and I cannot even begin to express my sincere gratitude for all of you.

Any questions, concerns or comments, let them rip … I will try to update as things progress.

Take Care and Much Love

Posted by Angels & HummingBirds & Fairies & CBear

at 6:04 PM

I still wrote in my journal for a few more days, usually while we were on the way to one appointment or another. It kept my mind busy and away from wondering to darker areas.

On October 7th I wrote the following in my journal: "We are headed to see the Surgeon to find out if we need another surgery— We shall see …"

I blogged the below later that day.

WEDNESDAY, OCTOBER 7, 2009

Well we just got back from seeing the surgeon and she said since there are still some abnormal cells in the lateral margin my choices are to either have a total mastectomy of the right breast or try and excise more of the lateral margin area. Since we are down to just one little area, I opted for the later. So the 3rd surgery, which will be the Charm, is scheduled for next Monday the 12th. After that then radiation, then chemo. My guess is chemo will not start before November now …

Next update will probably be the 13th.

Oh one other thing, if you want to still call, text or email that is fine. At least with this blog maybe we don't have to talk about my condition and I can hear how things are going for you.

Take Care and Thanks for being there for us! XOXOXOXOXO
Posted by Angels & HummingBirds & Fairies & CBear
at 9:12 AM

I also cancelled the appointment with the Radiation Oncology doctor's office. They would be call me back to reschedule.

On the morning of October 9th, I had a conversation and an epiphany so I blogged about it … I really liked blogging …

FRIDAY, OCTOBER 9, 2009

Positive Outlook
Hi All,

I was just emailing someone I keep in touch with through my work and decided some of the things I shared with her I wanted to share with everyone when it comes to my condition.

As I mentioned previously, my cousin has gone through something similar to what I am about to go through. We were talking about a week ago and my cousin is one of those people who sees the good in just about anything and through our discussion I came to realize I can look at what I am about to embark upon as an opportunity for a clean slate.

In other words, going through the surgeries, radiation and chemo is a very thorough, inside and out full body detoxification and insurance is paying for most of it. This situation has also made me take a look at how well I take care of myself.

Now those of you who know me would probably say I am pretty conscientious about my diet and I lean towards natural remedies vs. synthetic remedies. I try to exercise on a regular basis also. Even so, somehow a couple of cells decided to have a party in my right breast and create a little havoc. Well, diet and trying to exercise isn't the only factor when it comes to something like this. There is emotional well being. Emotional well being does not mean someone that can suck it up when times are tough. Emotional well being, as I have learned, is someone that can express themselves and let their emotions out as they arise. I have done a lot of sucking up and not afforded myself what I have suggested others afford themselves. If there is one thing I never thought I was, is a hypocrite. Eeesh, the things you find out about yourself when you really have to take a long look in the mirror. While I would never do anything intentional to hurt another human being, I have done just that by not taking total and proper care of myself emotionally. Well, no more of that passive irresponsible behavior.

To not allow yourself some me time is not good and I am all about good these days. I have committed to 2 hrs of me time daily. I can do whatever I want to do in those 2 hrs and it is all about me. I encourage everyone to do the same. You are going to have to make the time one way or the other and it doesn't have to be 2 hrs. Just commit some time daily to yourself. If you are a single parent and know another single parent, see if you all can work together to get that me time. I know someone who trains for marathons, I would imagine the times she is running, is her me time, and I will add this woman works very hard and long hours, but she manages to allow herself some me time and I don't recall her ever being really sick. Just so you know I consider writing in this blog me time. I am expressing my thoughts and reaching out to the people I care about. Hoping they will learn from my experiences. Next I am going to exercise for 30 minutes or as much as I can take and I will meditate. Then if I feel up to it and have a few minutes I will do something crafty, as I like

to be creative. So, maybe we should consider a Me time movement ...
What do you think!
Posted by Angels & HummingBirds & Fairies & CBear
at 8:01 AM

Later in the day, something phenomenal happened to me. I was driving west on Greenway, headed to the hospital to get another pre-op x-ray done. My thoughts were running wild. I was saddened by some regrets I had about things I didn't do that I should have done, things I did that I shouldn't have done, and mistakes I made raising my children. I was trying really hard to forgive myself. I told myself the past is in the past and all I could do was learn and go forward. It was a struggle but I continued to talk myself through it. In the midst of my thoughts, I noticed a black car with limo-tinted windows pass me at a moderate rate of speed on the right and merged in front of me. It wasn't aggressive, just noticeable. I was still trying to talk myself into forgiveness when we came upon a red light. This black car was stopped in front of me. All of a sudden, I saw some big white lettering on the rear window of the black car, and it said, "FORGIVEN," I kid you not. Right then and there I literally broke down in tears and said, "Thank you!" The light turned green and the car traveled another half a block and made a right-hand turn. After the x-ray, I called my cousin Susan and told her what had happened and started crying again. I definitely needed what I got at that moment. I sincerely believe we are getting messages all the time. We need to allow these messages to guide us. The memory of this, still tugs at my heart.

The day for surgery number three is upon us. Before we went I just had to blog ...

MONDAY, OCTOBER 12, 2009

Pre-3rd Surgery

Just about to leave to check in for this 3rd and final surgery. I say it that way because I am manifesting a positive outcome for this surgery. I have meditated this morning with the positive thought, "they are going to remove all of the cancerous cells all the cancerous cells will be gone!"

Hope you all have a good day! I will try to update tomorrow ... Take Care!

Posted by Angels & HummingBirds & Fairies & CBear
at 8:56 AM

The surgery prep was the same routine as the last two, but this time, in addition to the excision, the surgeon would place a port-a-cath on the left side of my chest about three inches down from my collar bone. I wanted to talk with the surgeon before surgery and let her know after everything is said and done that I was going to have breast reduction surgery, so take all the tissue she needed to take. I was a 36 DD and it just seemed like the more tissue you have, the more chance you have of having an issue. A part of me was also thinking that if I give the Surgeon this permission, maybe she would get it all for sure this time.

After surgery ... I thought she got it all this time. I felt it in my bones. All I could think at this point was that hopefully we can get on with this now. I just wanted to get this over and done with.

TUESDAY, OCTOBER 13, 2009

Post 3rd Surgery

Okay, I believe this 3rd and final excision surgery was the charm. I talked with the surgeon prior to the surgery to let her know I am planning on having a breast reduction to even things up. I am a Libra, I will go crazy if I am not balanced, seriously. So, in saying that I gave her all the latitude she needed to get all of the cancerous cells. The surgeon was out in 25 mins to speak with my husband and aunt, to which she told them, "I did well in surgery," she was very aggressive about the tissue she took, she went all the way to the skin line on the lateral side and she is confident we are going to have clear margins. She did have to extend the incision a bit, but that is okay I have some really good vitamin E to put on it. Prior to surgery, the surgeon told us she has asked the pathologist to look at the tissue STAT, and they should have the results by no later than 5pm on the 13th. I am scheduled to see the surgeon on the 14th 7 am for the results and have the balloon placed for Radiation.

Radiation

The plan is I will receive Brachytherapy radiation treatment. What is that, you may ask … Well, in a nutshell, or should I say in a balloon LOL, they insert a balloon into the cavity where the lump was removed. It is filled with saline, except the canal going through the center of the balloon which it has a catheter connected to it. The canal is where the radiation seed will be injected via the catheter via a computer twice a day. The time in between injecting the radiation seed is no less than 6 hours. This is done for 5 days in total. In my case with the balloon being placed this Wednesday, I will receive twice a day (BID) radiation seeds, Thursday, Friday, Monday, Tuesday, and Wednesday. So radiation should be done by October 21st afternoon. That is when they will take out the balloon.

So why choose this line of radiation treatment. Well, I am sure you have noticed the obvious, that being the duration of treatment. 5 days sure does beat the heck out of 5-7 weeks, 5 days a week external radiation treatment. The other advantage is the only cells affected are the ones that surrounded the lump. In other words not so many good cells are being radiated. Also, the amount of time for each administration is no more than 30 minutes and most of that is to set up and disconnect from the computer. What are the side effects? They are minimal compared to external radiation, but here are a few:

- Scar tissue
- Fat Necrosis (2% chance)
- Infection, this is always a possibility when a catheter is placed.

All in all, not too bad compared to other treatment options. I did hear from one patient in the Doctors office, she did have some burning of the skin, but this was done on her 5+ years prior and I am not sure they were using computers back then. The potential for uneven distribution of the radiation was higher if a computer was not used.

Well, I think that pretty much sums it up at this point. My next update will be on the 14th after the balloon has been placed. Please let me know if you have any questions and if you are reading this blog, think about being a follower and setting it so when a New post is entered it will notify you, so you know when to look for updates.

Take Care, Be Safe and Be True to Yourself ...

Posted by Angels & HummingBirds & Fairies & CBear
at 8:10 AM

The 14th begins on a good note.

WEDNESDAY, OCTOBER 14, 2009

Act 2 Scene 1

Okey dokey, we are now into Act 2, meaning the lateral margin came back clear, but we knew that was going to be the case didn't we.

Bright and early at 7 am the surgeon implanted the balloon as previously mentioned. I took a vicodin 30 mins prior and was given a local, so all I felt was a little pressure. I used to watch surgeries on TV so I am interested in what is going on when they are doing the procedures, so a local works for me. The surgeon filled the balloon with 50cc of saline, which filled the void and blew my breast right back up. It is kind of a funny sensation, sometimes if I move to quickly it's kind of like whoosh. It is kind of hard to explain, but it doesn't hurt. It is just different.

Next, I had to go get a CT scan from the Radiation Oncologists office to verify the placement of the balloon and give measurements to the Doctor and Physicist to make sure the correct dose of radiation is administered for the next 5 days of treatment. I have to go in to the facility at 8 or 8:30 am and 2:30 pm daily starting tomorrow until next Wednesday, with the weekend off. In addition to the CT scan the Radiation therapists measured the catheters and cut them down as needed. They also made sure the balloon is positioned correctly for administration.

No sleeping on the right side, sponge baths only, take an antibiotic until gone, no lifting any weight with my right arm, overall take it easy. For reassurance I asked about side effects and the Therapist told me it is rare that there are any side effects and most patients report a warm sensation, but otherwise not much else. I did ask about the woman who experienced burning 5 yrs ago. The therapist said this therapy has come a long way in the last 5 yrs.

I feel pretty good about this therapy and the Dr overseeing this seems to be a very good person. I have done some research on him and he is one of the best in his field, but more importantly I get the feeling he really cares about his patients. He presents as he is there to help you in a very sincere and caring manner.

Well, that is about it for today ... I am going to veg and take some me time. Over the next week I will blog as things progress or when it strikes me to do so.

Posted by Angels & HummingBirds & Fairies & CBear
at 1:05 PM

Blogging was my way of staying connected since it felt like I had been taken out of the mainstream of life ...

THURSDAY, OCTOBER 15, 2009

Act 2 Scene 2
There are a total of 10 treatments with this type of Radiation and as of 3 pm today I have completed 2 of them. The first one was at 8:30 am and the second was at 2:30 pm.

When I get there they take me into an office and do an ultrasound to make sure the balloon is as it should be. They also extract any air and/or fluid that has built up in the cavity. Next I am taken into the room where they hook 4 of the 5 catheters up to a machine that is set to deliver a certain dosage of radiation over a certain duration of time, depending on the measurements taken from the CT scan done yesterday. Other than a slight discomfort from the catheters protruding from my body and a balloon in my breast, no side effects have presented themselves. The Physicist did tell me I will probably start feeling very tired after the 3rd day of treatment, which will be next Monday.

I am scheduled to see the Oncologist next Tuesday the 20th. Since I will still be getting radiation at this time I did contact the Oncologist's office and explained to them I will still be doing radiation and do they still want me to come in, but not necessarily to get treatment. I did talk with the Radiation Oncologist about this and he said the Oncologist probably doesn't realize the delay due to the 3rd surgery. He said to go on in and let the Doctor know I am still getting radiation. It is on the way home anyway, so we will stop in.

So, Tuesday is going to be a pretty full day. Radiation at 8:30 am, Oncologist 9:00 am or when we get there, more like 9:30, then radiation again at 2:30 pm.

As I was getting my treatments today I was thinking about how wonderful my house is going to look someday when we get it remodeled. I was mostly thinking about the front patio I want to create. The flooring will be flagstone with low growing herbs growing between them. Then there will be slats for the roof, so the sun and rain could get through. I want some climbing plants to grow up the poles and through the roof. We will hang the swing from the roof and have a fire pit in the corner furthest from the house. I also want a 3' fence around the patio and a small water flowing device to promote calmness and relaxation. Can't wait until it is done, but until then I will go there in my mind and it will come to be.

Well until the next posting, take it easy and think happy thoughts! Hasta …

Posted by Angels & HummingBirds & Fairies & CBear
at 4:23 PM

Here is a journal entry from October 18th: "I received a message from the Radiation Oncology doctor's office; not to go in for my appointment on the 19th because the radiation machine had an issue. They would call me with a time when they sorted things out."

My last journal entry was on October 19th: "I received a call from the Radiation Oncology doctor's office this morning. They said, they would do 1 treatment today and make up the missed treatment on Thursday. Bummer! That meant I needed to sleep one more night with this balloon in me. It felt like my boob had morphed into an alien or octopus ..."

I had a bit of a mental breakdown this morning. It had been building up for a couple of days. It helped to get it out because I had a feeling of despair like I wanted to give up and die. I felt so conflicted because I tried to maintain my belief that everything happened for a reason. There is no such thing as coincidences, yet I still felt hopelessness. I talked to Ric about how I was feeling and told him I was okay with dying. I have loved and been loved, for that I am grateful and would die a happy woman. I had forgiven myself and others and believed when I did pass on, I would be with Kaity, Lorie, my grandparents, and friends that have passed.

It's funny because everyone said I had such a positive attitude ... Wow, I didn't realize I could be so good at being one way on the outside and completely opposite on the inside. I always thought I wore my heart on my sleeve. As I worked through these emotions, I came to the conclusion that this might be happening because Kaity's Way is where I was to focus my attention. I should have faith in what we are doing, as well as in myself, to grow Kaity's Way. You see, I wasn't willing to take the sacrificial leap to Kaity's Way for fear of not making it and causing financial issues for the family.

Well now I felt as if I had no choice. I needed to flow with this, my thoughts told me, one should not doubt themselves.

TUESDAY, OCTOBER 20, 2009

Act 2 Scene 3

Well here we are a little more than midway through Radiation. There was a hiccup yesterday as there was a software issue detected with the Radiation machine and my Monday morning appointment was canceled. So, I only had 1 treatment yesterday in the afternoon.

This morning we went in for my 6th radiation treatment and then the Oncologist afterwards. Because I am in the midst of Radiation the Chemo has been postponed. I will start chemo on 10/29/09. I was really hoping with all the delays some other type of therapy rose as an option, Nope not this time.

After my treatment yesterday we stopped by the Moon Valley plant nursery on Thunderbird, it is closing so they are having a liquidation sale. I went in there to see what they had, but found myself walking around enjoying being in an environment filled with so much life and energy. I didn't buy anything, but really enjoyed being around all the plants and hearing the birds. I feel as if I had absorbed some of the positive energy given off by the plants. I felt good after being there. I am going to stop and walk through again today, just to get that energy lift. My last treatment is Thursday morning, so I will probably pick up some plants to put in the yard. I love to garden and watch things grow, but haven't been taking the time to do so in the last couple of years. I think I am going to take this situation as an opportunity to get back to doing the things I love.

You know more me time ...

As of this Thursday around 9 am, I am going to be free of this balloon and take some time to heal from where the balloon is removed before Chemo starts. I am going to take it easy and relax. Maybe I will focus on some preemptive healing before we get this party started.

Until next time, I hope everything in your world is filled with Love, joy and positive energy.

Take care and be good to yourself!

Posted by Angels & HummingBirds & Fairies & CBear

at 12:02 PM

I really did like the oncologist. He always asked if we needed anything from him. We were so new to this that we had yet to say yes. I needed to think of a reason to say yes so that I could engage him in further conversation. He was so somber but seemed to have had a bit of a twinkle in his eye. It was as if he had hope yet tried to keep it tucked away for fear of what may happen. I bet he was absolutely brilliant. Next visit I decided I would ask him about his horses. That should get us started.

SATURDAY, OCTOBER 24, 2009

End of Act 2

Well as of 10/21/09 ~9 am the Balloon was removed and radiation is done. What a relief, but I am glad I had this option for radiation 5 days BID vs 5 x wk for 7 wks. Other than being energy drained and having a foreign object sticking out of your body, there were no other side effects for me. On the bright side I learned how to sleep on my back, less wrinkles. I used to be a belly or right side sleeper.

What's next, well now I am preparing for the chemotherapy, which is to begin October 29th 9:30 am. I am told the treatment time frame is 3 hours, so we should be done around 12:30pm. I have done some research, couldn't help myself, and found there are a couple of things I can do to prepare my body inside and out for the side effects of chemotherapy. From what I understand, the drugs used for chemotherapy target the fast growing cells which are found in your digestive track, mouth, skin, bottoms of your feet, palm of your hands and hair follicles. They target the fast growing cells because that is what abnormal cells are, fast growing.

I have been ingesting 30 gms of L-Glutamine daily. It's tasteless and adds some texture to whatever you are drinking. If you drink it with water it is kind of like drinking very diluted baking soda water. Almost like flat soda water. I add it to orange juice, soy milk, smoothies, green tea. Not bad at all. I have also been taking Aloe Vera Shooters 3 x a day. I have tried Papaya orange and Cherry Berry, neither one masks the flavor of the aloe vera very well, but it is tolerable so long as it is just an ounce at a time. Both the L-Glutamine and Aloe Vera will help my digestive track when the chemotherapy drugs attack it. Hopefully I will have less nausea and, eeesh, diarrhea.

Often times mouth sores will develop. To keep this to a minimum my aunt suggested I eat a popsicle while the drugs are being administered. She said this did work for her. We have a package of popsicles all ready to take with us on the 29th. There is also a baking soda rinse you can do as a follow up for mouth sores.

For the skin, drinking plenty of water daily, 4 to 5 16.9 oz bottles should be good. I have been trying to make sure I get at least 4 drank by end of day. This is in addition to juice (oj, apple), green tea (hot in the morning & cold with my lunch). Then it is recommended you moisturize twice a day with an unscented good moisturizing lotion head to toe. We got Aveeno and Goldbond with Shea Butter. My cousin suggested the Shea Butter, the thicker the better. For my face I have good ole Oil of Olay or a knock off, gotta save those pennies LOL

Now for the bottom of my feet and palm of my hands; My aunt and I are going to go out and get some gloves for my hands and booties for my feet and some aloe vera gel I will put on my hands and feet then put the gloves and booties on, during treatment. I bought some pajamas from Ross that match my purple slippers, I plan to wear to each chemo treatment. The funny thing is the shirt of the pajamas is Breast Cancer Pink and the pants are polka dotted and some of them are purple that is how I tied the slippers in. With that said, I will have to make sure the gloves and booties are color coordinated of course. The pajamas were only $12.99 and once chemotherapy is over, I am going to burn them as another chapter ending in celebration of a new beginning.

So, now for the hair follicles, well as far as I can tell, there really is not much that can be done to avoid the losing of hair. Some people lose all their hair; others only lose the hair on their head, but will retain their eyebrows and eyelashes. Some people have commented on the positive side as the hair on your legs falls out so no need to shave. Who knows what will happen to me. I am not much for wigs, but will probably get one just to have on hand just in case. I think I am going to go to a wig shop this next week before my treatment so they can evaluate and maybe put something together with my current hair style. I am not sure if I am going to shave my head or just get it cut like Jamie Lee Curtis has hers done in the Activia commercial. I'm not sure my hair will lay like hers because her hair *looks to be on the fine side. If it doesn't lay right I will just spike it. Ahhhh who cares, it's only hair. It will grow back eventually and maybe very different from what fell out. My aunt's hair came back about the same color, but is not quite as thick as it was. My cousin's hair was a dark blonde shade, straight and thick but fine strands. Her hair came back a chestnut color, very wavy and thick. That just goes to show you there may be little change or lots of change. After my hair falls out, I see myself wearing head wraps and the like. With us coming into the winter months, hats and head wraps are in. I have also considered getting a henna tattoo on my head. I am thinking something with Angels, hummingbirds, fairies and my husband and children's names. I am sure that is pretty pricey so I may not indulge. It's just a thought.*

A part of me is scared, but then I am okay with what I have to do to rid myself of any possibility of abnormal cells floating around in my body. There are worse things in life than this, so I am trying not to be too much of a baby about this.

I am concerned about my husband as he is my primary caregiver and often times situations such as this are just as hard on the caregiver as it is on the patient. He is trying to do everything right and work on top of it, I am very fortunate and count my blessings every day to have such an unconditionally loving and caring man in my life. When I was going for the Radiation treatments he went to all but one with me. Then I noticed there was a woman that came to her treatments alone every day, we were on the same schedule, and she was the appt after me for each treatment. She was a nice lady and who knows maybe she preferred to go to her appts alone. All I know is I was glad that my husband was with me every time I went.

Well, that is about all for now. If I feel up to it I will blog shortly after my treatment, if not, I will eventually blog, because I just can't seem to help myself. I think I might write a book.

Tootaloo, ciao, hasta la vista, until the next time …

Posted by Angels & HummingBirds & Fairies & CBear

at 8:39 PM

THURSDAY, OCTOBER 29, 2009

Act 3 Scene 1

Okay I made it to the facility for my first chemo treatment. I am prepared, I believe. I have been drinking so much water, juice and green tea that I am afraid I am going to float away. I have also been lotioning up twice a day with Aveeno and Gold Bond Shea Butter lotions and this morning I stuck to the toilet seat. Whoops! Okay maybe TMI, but it made you giggle, right? I told my husband and let him know since this happened he now has a new duty… Make sure when I come out of public restrooms I don't have any of those paper seat protectors hanging out of my backside … How embarrassing!

We saw the Doctor first, everything looks good and he explained he is going to give me some samples of an anti nausea drug and a RX for decadron to get filled. It is also an anti nausea drug.

When we walked into the treatment area the first thing I eye spied was a seat I could look out a window and I sit down. The blinds are closed so I will have to ask them to open them. Not sure if the other patients will be okay with this. There are 5 people here getting their treatments. One lady is by herself and very much keeps to herself, then there are two men who appear friendly. One is very cold and covered up with 3 blankets. The other man is very personable and smiles a lot. Next to him is a woman who is very quiet but smiles (she is asleep now). Next to her there is another woman listening to her ipod and seems to enjoy it. A new lady just walked in and sat across from the lady I first spoke of and they are chatting it up. The first lady I spoke of appears to have been through a few treatments already and if I am not mistaken she said this is her last treatment. She has been talking with the new lady and from the sound of the conversation the new lady is new to this, maybe one treatment under her belt. She still has her hair, but mentioned some was coming out, but not like bald spot clumps. The lady that is on her last treatment was explaining some stuff to the new lady ... A little camaraderie, cool beans!

Well back to me, so far they have put the catheter in the port, taken blood for a CBC they will do right here in the office and more blood will be sent out for a CMP to make sure my potassium and the like are in check. The nurse said the port looked really good and was working good. Before she tapped the port she sprayed some freezing stuff, so it would be painless and it was. The nurse offered us a 2 for 1 deal, but my husband passed ... Hmmmmm I wonder why. I would have passed to if I had the option. I do, but I also don't want to have the worry of cancer floating around in my blood day in and day out.

The nurse is here again she has hung some bags on the IV pole with benadryl, aloxy, tagamet, dexamethasone this is all for anti nausea and to make sure I don't have an allergic reaction. At the end of treatment I will be given a shot of Neulasta which could cause some bone discomfort it is a histamine so it is suggested I take claritin and tylenol for any discomfort. This drug is a long lasting bone marrow booster so my white count does not plummet leaving me open for infections. The nurse also *gave me the sample anti nausea, Anzemet and told me the RX for the Decadron is in my blue folder. I didn't know I had one, but I guess that will be explained later. She also gave me some literature on the Neulasta and why they do a CBC. The benadryl is being administered now, so I am going to put this away for now and come back to it later... feeling a little whoopy if you know what I mean ...*

After coming out of the whoopiness, I am pretty much doing fine. I do have a headache that doesn't seem to want to go away. I took tylenol about an hour ago and it is still there. I also feel exhausted, very fatigued. They gave me the 3 drugs in this order Cyclophosphamide 20 mg SDV Quantity 880 mg IV drip, then Taxotere 20 mg 40mg/ml IV drip, then the red one Adrimyacin 90 mg IV push. So, I am going to call it a night and just veg. Not sure what tomorrow will bring, but I will just flow with it.

Posted by Angels & HummingBirds & Fairies & CBear
at 5:31 PM

RJ's 24th Birthday was November 11th ... We skyped with him to wish him a Happy Birthday and talked with him for a bit. Since I was losing my hair, I wore a towel on my head like I had just gotten out of the shower. He was doing well even though he didn't much care for being in Korea. He made some great friends in the military and for that I am very thankful. His roommate walked by and saw me in the computer and said, "Nice towel." Ric and I just laughed given what we knew. It was not easy keeping this from RJ, but it was for his own good; that's what I kept telling myself. We had always tried to be open with our children, but I didn't see any good coming from him knowing about my condition at this time.

FRIDAY, NOVEMBER 13, 2009

Back in the Game

Well it has been a while since my last blog, because I spent most of the time in bed up until the 8th of November. Basically after the treatment once I went to bed I stayed in bed. My energy level was non-existent for several days. On the night of the 3rd I did not sleep a wink due to severe abdominal pain. I had been hot to the touch, but when I took my temperature it was only registering 99.3. I was also clammy and very very uncomfortable. It felt as if my system was shutting down on me and there was not a single thing I could do. My husband tried to contact the Oncologist, but their office did not open until after 9 am, so he contacted the Radiation Oncologist, who suggested we get some colace, drink lots of fluids and be sure to get in contact with Oncologist as it sounded like I might be getting the flu. Not good, the flu could throw things way off as far as my treatments go. I was very weak and was not capable of taking care of myself by myself for anything. Thank God for my husband, he is the best. He ended up calling into work and got a hold of the Oncologists office. What seemed like the end for me, came back as this is par for the course. My body was mad at me because I was not able to eliminate the toxins from the chemotherapy, the cells the chemotherapy had killed and the food I had eaten. Honestly speaking, I was ready to throw in the towel at this point. I have to say I give props to anyone that has gone through chemotherapy. This stuff is not just difficult; it is downright brutal. After a few days of being on a liquid diet and more pity parties than I really care to admit to, my system finally regulated and the 8th was the first day I had some pep in my step. Oh, there was one other symptom that arose after my system regulated, Indigestion. The kind that makes you feel like you are having a heart attack. I took Gas-X to remedy the indigestion. All of this made me scared to eat solid foods. It took a couple of days before I would chance solid food. I had absolutely no idea just how many food commercials are on TV. Arriba's is the one I saw the most. I was ready to scream every time I saw a food commercial. So then I started watching the Food Network. Not sure what I was thinking, but I got past the fear of eating solid food and I am on a regular diet now with lots of greens.

What did I learn from this … I went on a field trip one day with my aunt to Trader Joes and bought several types of creamy soups to eat after my next treatment. My cousin sent me a book called Green Smoothies, which we will pick a few to make for me to eat after my treatments. Yes, it is a liquid diet for me after my treatments up to 10 days post. We will find out if that will help with making sure my system flows regularly. I have Gas-X and Colace on hand just in case.

Posted by Angels & HummingBirds & Fairies & CBear
at 8:47 PM

I asked the oncologist about his horses and he cracked a smile. It seemed as though they were his release, his joy in life. I completely understood how that could be. I find horses to be magnificent animals and simply wonderful to be around. I would love to get back to horseback riding again someday. It would be awesome to have a horse someday (something for the bucket list). Yes, I was creating a bucket list for life. Yes, I was going to list out all the things I wanted to do and do them, more on that later.

The oncologist asked me what I did for a living, probably because I left a brochure in his office a couple of times by now.

I explained Kaity's Way and let him know I am on a mission and my work was not done yet, so I was going to beat this thing. As I was saying this, he held my chart close to his chest, like he was hugging it, and looked directly at me. I had his full undivided attention and that was nice. After I finished what I was saying, I saw a twinkle in his eye. To me that was him saying, you go girl! It was very encouraging. He of all people knew that people who had something to live for do not give up.

FRIDAY, NOVEMBER 13, 2009, continued

Next Symptom
My hair has been coming out. Yesterday about 75% of my hair came out. Oddly enough, there is still plenty of hair on my head to get by. My husband says if you have no idea how thick my hair was you would not know I was losing my hair. It is a very odd feeling to run your fingers through your hair and find most of it in the palm of your hand. So, my husband and I took a field trip to the American Cancer Society today. They are very nice people and gave me a complementary wig, scarf, hat and beanie. I am not so sure about the wig. My husband said I look like Meg Ryan in it. He is sweet … I tried it on again after we got home and I am not so sure I like it. I have to take it in to get it styled better; the bangs are too long for me. I am not even sure I will ever really wear it. I am more of a scarf/hat person. I figured it wouldn't be a bad idea to have one just in case. I have to say I like the hat the best. It is black and white hounds tooth. I thought I could wear a scarf or headband under it to add some color. The beanie is cool too. It is colorful and fuzzy. We then went to Walmart where we bought more scarves, headbands and gloves, so I don't have

to fist bump everyone who wants to shake my hand. I am pretty sure we will be doing a buzz cut on my hair within the next couple of days, because I really don't like finding my hair everywhere. The key to pulling this off is accessorizing. Time to get creative, which is my middle name ... With everything we got today and what my cousin sent me, I believe I am set for a while.

Posted by Angels & HummingBirds & Fairies & CBear
at 9:19 PM

Another thing about that day was my dear friend Denise was coming out for a visit from California. As I mentioned previously, we have been friends for many years and I love her. Even though we lived six hours away by car, when the chips are down, she has always been there for me. The last time I saw her was when Kaity passed. She came out and spent a few days with me to make sure I was okay. She is such a great friend and I a true blessing for me. Ric had gone to pick Denise up from the airport. I did not go because I was trying to stay away from populated places so I would not get sick.

We had a wonderful weekend. Believe it or not, while Denise was here, we had a fundraising yard sale for Kaity's Way, and she was a great help, no surprise there. Her and my Aunt Janie got along very well and went gaga over that game, Simon. Denise and I also went to Clarkdale, a town about 90 minutes north of Phoenix, to see a play called the MENding Monologues—a very good play by the way. We also had dinner at a Mexican restaurant and drove back home after the play. We also went to Dillard's Outlet to shop. They have some smoking deals and it was right by the house. Denise bought so much she had to pay an additional $50 to the airline for her bag being overweight on her return trip. Before Denise left, we put on an early Thanksgiving dinner. Mainly because my next treatment was scheduled a week before Thanksgiving and I knew I would not feel up to putting on or participating in a Thanksgiving dinner. We also wanted to include Denise in our dinner. It was a very nice and quiet dinner. That weekend made me forget I was a cancer patient. I really hated seeing Denise go. I wished we lived down the way from each other again. Nonetheless, as always, we would keep in touch, and we did.

FRIDAY, NOVEMBER 20, 2009

Bald is not only Beautiful, it is Liberating

Well as of last Saturday afternoon 11/14/09 I am bald. It was either that or walk around with the witchy poo look which was just too unbecoming. So, as my hair was continuing to come out as I was showering I grabbed a pair of scissors and started cutting at what was left of my hair. Then I got out of the shower and took the electric clippers to my head. I did all this by myself while my husband was picking my very dear friend, Denise, up at the airport. To lessen the surprise I texted my husband and told him I shaved my head. Then when they got home I took the towel off immediately to show them and said, "I just don't know what to do with my hair." We all laughed and I hugged Denise.

After a few days of wearing scarfs and hats I had gotten from the American Cancer Society and Walmart, I am getting used to this new look and liking it. It's all about the accessories ... I also like the bald look as weird as that may sound. I believe if it were warmer I would just go without a scarf or hat. I actually like my bald look. I even texted

a picture of myself to about 20 people. I am not photogenic so they will
have to see me in person to really appreciate the look.

Posted by Angels & HummingBirds & Fairies & CBear
at 11:14 AM

A new thing was happening to me when I was out and about, sporting my new look. Former cancer patients were acknowledging me. At first, it was kind of strange. People would just walk up to me and ask, "How long?" or "How many treatments have you had or have left?" They always had a look of empathy on their faces, so I would graciously answer. They would usually then speak words of encouragement and/or share their journey. There was one lady in Clarkdale, who approached me and asked how long I had been in treatment. I told her and she explained only a few years back she had battled cancer for the third time, the first time being over 20 years ago. She appeared to be about 20 years my senior, but to look at her, I would not have guessed she was a former cancer patient, let alone three times over. She appeared to have had a positive disposition, and I truly appreciated her sharing her experiences with me. All blessings…

FRIDAY, NOVEMBER 20, 2009, *continued*

1/3 of the way through Chemo

Yesterday was my 2nd Chemo treatment. My WBC and RBC were low,
but my platelets were up. I was put on the same regimen of drugs all
the way to the Nuelasta. I was discussing my WBC and RBC numbers
with the nurses to find out if there is anything I can do to help the
number and they gave me a really cool cook book that has recipes for

dishes by symptom. So, after I get through the first 10 days of the liquid diet, I will ease into the recipes in this cook book. I have been looking for something like this since I was approaching my 1st treatment, so I am very glad to have it.

Yesterday after treatment we went shopping and I was a bit wiped out after that. I also had a headache and experienced some nausea. I was reluctant to take the anti-nausea drug (compazine) as one of the side effects is constipation. That word just scares me, but my wonderful intelligent husband suggested I take the compazine with a colace and it worked. No constipation today, but when I got up this morning my face was very red in color for about an hour and has calmed down since. I just asked my husband if it were still red, but her dee dur I have on a red beanie, so I guess it wouldn't look all that red. I took the beanie off and asked my daughter who said my cheeks are still pink in color. It also feels warm to the touch for me. Overall I feel pretty okay today. Who knows what tomorrow will bring, I am just thankful for the good days at this point.

One other thing, I am under 150 pounds. I weighed in at 148.5, yippee. I wonder how much of that was hair?

Until the next time—Take Care!

Posted by Angels & HummingBirds & Fairies & CBear
at 11:31 AM 0 comments

FRIDAY, NOVEMBER 27, 2009

SOUP, is not for me!

Okay, I really tried the liquid diet idea for about 1 ½ days and just couldn't do it any longer. To say, think, hear or spell the word SOUP, puts a lump in my throat and gives me a slight nausea sensation. It really takes me a minute to get over it. I use the word stew to get me through the day now. I don't know what happened in my brain, but I just can't do or say it anymore. Now I did stay on liquids for about a day and a half more, just water and apple/prune juice.

I think part of the issue was a film I would get in my mouth, which no matter how much you brush your teeth or swish, it is there and gives everything a funky taste.

Then there is the reason for the liquid diet, which was to avoid constipation. Well it didn't work. While most of the people who shared their experiences with me had diarrhea after treatment, I just have to be the complete opposite. Since, even being on a liquid diet for 3 days and still having problems with constipation, I have pretty much decided this is par for the course for me after treatment. I haven't quite figured out what I am going to try next to avoid it for the next treatment, but I will come up with something.

It's Crazy that for the last 8 days my whole life revolved around the possibility of a good POOP! For crying out loud, I am only 46 years old and I was praying daily for a good POOP! I didn't pray for good luck, prosperity, my health, others or their health all I wanted to do was POOP. I drank prune/apple juice, took 400 mg of a stool softener daily, drank as much water as I could, took apple cider vinegar tablets, and finally succumbed to suppositories and nothing, nada, nunc, zero POOP production, just plenty of indigestion.

Here is my conclusion on what my digestive/intestinal track is doing. It is plain and simply revolting against me. They are saying, "You are putting toxins in us and you expect us to perform as usual, nothing doing." Another thing they are saying is, "You are just gonna have to wait until we are ready, so chill out we will let you know when we are ready to start moving again!" It makes sense, but what an inconvenience. At least this time around there was not so much pain involved. I think it is due to being on a liquid diet for 3 days. I also think doing everything we did helped also, just not as fast as I would have liked. Nonetheless, I am back on track pooping better as of today and will hopefully stay that way until my next treatment. At least now I can pray for more than POOP!

Posted by Angels & HummingBirds & Fairies & CBear
at 9:51 AM

SUNDAY, DECEMBER 13, 2009

It's been a while and life goes on...

Yes indeed, life does go on... It's funny, because every time I turn around I am reminded in one way or another I am a person fighting breast cancer. Every time I look in the mirror I see the bump (port) on the left side of my chest or my bald head. Then there is when I am getting dressed to go out somewhere, I have to consider what hat or scarf I am going to wear to match my clothes. Then when I am out, there is the constant concern about my headgear slipping. The thought kind of makes me chuckle, but I worry more about freaking other people out. Besides knowing me like I do, it is bound to happen at least once, I just hope it is around someone who will get a good laugh out of it, rather than be scarred for life.

Oh, but life does go on ... One day you're minding your own business, trying to get some errands ran before your next treatment. After getting home from grocery shopping on a stormy day, you find your electricity is out. The transformer behind the house has blown a breaker, and because this is not the first time you know, you better get on the phone with APS or they will never know. The last time this happened was in July 2008 and we were without electricity for nearly 24 hours only to find out after 20 hours of no electricity APS never knew we were without electricity. For some reason it did not show on their grid. So needless to say, we do not think it will just come back on eventually. While on the phone with APS I let them know there was a big boom behind the house and it sounded like the transformer behind us blew again. Within 2 hours the lights are coming back on around us, but not for us or our next door neighbor and next door to them. Back on the phone again with APS, letting them know we still do not have power and we really need power due to my condition. An hour later I get a call from APS asking if our power is back on. I tell them no and they direct me to turn off all my circuit breakers and turn them back on. Okay, now they are pushing it, because I have been zapped far too many times to appreciate dealing with electricity in any way, nonetheless, my family needs me so tada ta ... da I proceed with turning off all the circuit breakers, knowing any minute now I am going to find myself 3 houses down and scorched. At least I don't have any hair to turn into an afro, LOL! All circuit breakers off wait 10 seconds now turn them back on ... All of them turn on except the main circuit breaker. Dog gone it, it won't hold in the on position ... Eeeesh! Now I have really done it.

Thank goodness our neighbor is an electrician, so I have him come over and confirm I am not just being a wimp and the main circuit breaker is really messed up. He does confirm the main circuit breaker is really messed up. Oh joy at least I am not a whimp ... lol.

What next ... now I have to tell my husband what I have done, he is cool about it and we get APS out to let us know what we need to do. They put some plastic tags on our electrical box and explain we need to get a new main circuit breaker. Our neighbor tries to track one down, mind you it is around 4:30 pm on a Monday, so everyone that sells electrical supplies are closed or are closing shortly and none are in our part of town. So, we have to wait until the next day to start our search. Temperatures are in the 30's and 40's due to the storm so we pack up some belongings and with kids and dogs in tow head to a local hotel/ motel for warm shelter.

The next day my husband goes to the electrical supply store first thing in the morning to find out they do not have one in stock, but can order it (our house is nearly 50 yrs old), and it will be in the next morning at 10:30. Next morning is much better than next week. So we are held up another night in the hotel/motel. Now because check out is at 11 am, we pay for 2 more nights. We needed somewhere to be, dogs and all, until the electricity came back on. Not to mention our neighbor would put the breaker in, but didn't get off work until 3pm. Incidentally, our two neighbors' electricity did come back on Monday night around 7 pm. The APS guy said had I not kept calling in, they would not have known we were down after everyone else in the neighborhood came back up. It can pay off to be a pest and a pest I can be ...

After my husband lets me know we will be in the hotel/motel for probably 2 more nights I go to the house and check on things and then work out a plan for the refrigerator and freezer food. Another neighbor, bless her heart, was able to clear 2 shelves in her refrigerator and 3 in her freezer so we could save our food. I would say, she helped save at least $150 in food. It is so nice to have such Great neighbors. I have to say during such a trying time the people around us really pulled together and helped us out.

By Wednesday evening we had the electricity back on, but the house was freezing and we were all so exhausted we just closed up the house and went back to the hotel/motel to sleep.

Looking back on things we were reminded what wonderful neighbors we have as well as it could have been worse. You see, my 3rd treatment was scheduled for the Thursday after we got back into the house. So, after treatment I was able to go home and start the healing process all over again. The timing would have been really bad had the power went out on Tuesday or Wednesday. So, that is why it has been a while ... I am starting to fade now, so I will try to blog tomorrow on how I am feeling since my 3rd treatment. Take Care!

Posted by Angels & HummingBirds & Fairies & CBear

at 3:16 PM

The upside of December 13th was that it's our oldest daughter Yvonne's 26th Birthday. She came over for a bit and we just sat around and talked. I wasn't much in the party mood, but I had never let anything get in the way of one of my kids' birthdays. Celebrating the birth of a child is a great day. I feel very blessed to be the mother of five. Yes, I say five even though I only gave birth to three. While Dan and Kaity did not grow in my womb, they did grow in my heart. Who says you had to be biologically related to someone to love them as much if not more than yourself?

MONDAY, DECEMBER 14, 2009

Halfway Done!!!!

My 3rd treatment was Dec 10 and it kicked my butt from the get go ... I am sure I felt myself tank about half way through it. I am not sure what that is all about, but usually I had about 2 days after treatment before I faded to chemo land, not this time. I could barely handle a little grocery shopping on the way home. When we got home, to bed it was for me. It was as if my energy level went through the floor. My appetite went right along with it. I mean I wanted nothing to eat or drink. I just wanted to fade away until it passed. I do have a couple of theories though. It is possible I overdid it with the power going out and all and exhausted myself. It could also be that the dreaded cumulative affect I have heard of has crept up on me. I can only control the first theory, so I will try real hard not to overdo it before my next treatment.

Oh and then the worst thing happened this time around. I vomited Saturday night. It just came out of nowhere. I don't recall having a pre-nausea feeling just that blasted film in my mouth. I was rinsing the film out of my mouth and that is when it happened. Gross! I was appalled. Then I couldn't stop. I am one of those people when someone vomits, I join the party if I don't get out of there. Needless to say my husband did vomit detail with the kids, because I could not stomach it. I wasn't stomaching my own. I just could not get away from myself. If anyone wanted to get away from themselves it was me at that very moment. Had my husband not showed up to console me I probably would have gone out of my mind!

The next day I realized my husband, bless his heart, took inventory of what I vomited. Only because I had asked for some maalox or mylanta to help with indigestion and he said I am not so sure about that, I believe you threw it up last night. No maalox or mylanta for me, only the pink stuff. The indigestion is relentless this time around also. Before all of this I was a gas bag. I had no idea it could be worse and burn so much. I am sure the vomiting has exacerbated this also.

The upside, my pooper seems to be working just fine for the time being. Thank goodness for that. Also, because my daughter has to pull shower detail, her and I have some really cool conversations about life. I really enjoy those moments with her. My mommy came over today to make us dinner and hang out with me. So, I got to spend time with my mommy also. The way I see it, my daughter got mommy time, I got daughter and mommy time and my mommy got daughter time, how cool is that!

Until next time, take care and if I do not blog before the 25th I wish everyone the Happiest of Holidays and a Great New Year!

Posted by Angels & HummingBirds & Fairies & CBear

at 5:53 PM

The vomiting must have really caused me to tailspin because I began to think, "I am done." No more, no mas, I was not doing this anymore ... I kept this to myself, but I was seriously contemplating telling the doctor that I wasn't going to do any more treatments. It was just too much. As I was thinking this through, Yvonne called me and said, "My friend said you need to finish all your treatments then everything will be fine." How the heck did he and she do that? I was so blown away by that phone call. I had not verbalized my thoughts to anyone. They were really starting to freak me out, but in a good way. The only thing I could think was my sister Lorie or maybe my grandmother or Nana was tapping into this person, who I had never met, to relay messages to me. All I knew at this point was once again I was being guided, so I needed to allow myself to be led.

TUESDAY, DECEMBER 15, 2009

A New Side Effect

I forgot to mention yesterday, there is one more new side effect I have been experiencing with round 3. I am crying a lot since the 3rd treatment. It is bizarre for me to be so emotional.

I mean I am normally an emotional passionate person, but this is beyond emotional. In the past if I cried it was usually due to frustration or complete and utter sadness. Okay there were also times if the right music was playing with a movie or commercial I would tear up, but that was usually when I was PMSing. Now what I am experiencing is crying at the thought of certain things, even sometimes at what feels like the drop of a dime. For instance how sad a friend of mine was when she found out about my condition. It just breaks my heart how sad she had become. The other day I was just lying in my bed crying and not even sure why, but I was boo hooing it big time.

The other day my sister in law called to find out how I was doing and to talk with me. She had said she was praying for me and the water works started. Maybe I was overwhelmed because she has the hook up, she is an Ordained Minister. Until my diagnosis my sister in law and I respected each other and have a love for the same man, but we really did not have much to do with each other. When we got together, which hasn't been often, she lives in Texas, we had a good time. Don't get me wrong there were no ill feelings just no opportunity to get to know each other over the last 18 years. Even so, since my diagnosis, she has been right by our sides doing what she can to comfort us. I say us, because I know it does my husband's heart good to know she is there. Not that she would have it any other way; because since

I met her I could see she and my husband had a solid sibling love for each other. They have a closeness that no matter if they only speak once a year they don't seem to miss a thing. When they are together a person can totally see they love each other and would be there for each other no matter what, and they are.

I don't really know where all these tears are coming from, but oddly enough, most times I feel a sense of relief. Maybe this is my body's way of get rid of some of the drugs. Or maybe I just need to learn how to feel for real. The Doctor did say chemo could throw me into menopause, so maybe the emotion is coming from there. Personally, I think it is a combination of all. Actually, I am okay with the emotion coming through. I feel more alive these days, and it has been a while since I have felt this alive. I am thinking I fell into somewhat of a depression nearly 2 yrs ago and have not done much to escape it. My sister, God rest her soul, tried to pull me out of it, but she was gone before I made it out.

It makes a person wonder, since I believe everything happens for a reason. Is the reason for me being on this journey to wake me up and realize where I was is no place for someone to reside? It is time for me to realize living is a gift and I need to respect that and live each day to the fullest? You know what they say, tomorrow is not guaranteed, so make the best of today.

Until next time Ciao …

Posted by Angels & HummingBirds & Fairies & CBear
at 1:32 PM

Tis the season, so I decided to bake some cookies to lift my spirits. I pulled out some simple recipes and started baking. They had to be simple because baking is not something I was very good at in the past. I found baking, unlike cooking, required you to follow a recipe to the letter. Those that knew what they were doing could probably vary from the recipe and be successful, but I learned there is some serious chemistry involved with baking.

One strange thing I did while going through treatment was I got hooked on watching the food channels. I watched just about every cooking show that was on the air. I'm not quite sure what I was thinking. For some reason, I found it very interesting and enjoyed learning about cooking and baking. Was I a glutton for punishment? Who knew?

I do not recall how many dozens of cookies I made, but we had cookies coming out of our ears. I have a tendency to do that when I get started on something. I'm not sure what I was thinking, but then it occurred to me that I could give them away for the holidays. Given that my income was cut in half, we did not have much money to put presents under the tree. This was a great way to tell my friends and family how much we loved and appreciated them. I put some in some tins and labeled them for friends and family. Then Heidi called me and told me she wanted to come over to visit after work and I was more than happy to have the company. More spirit lifting!

Heidi, true to her word showed up later that day, and was a sight for sore eyes. She had a basket of cookies for me and my family from the cookie exchange they did at work. Everyone that participated brought in enough for all the participants and me. How cool was that? And how cool was it that I had a bunch of cookies I baked to send back with Heidi? That was such a nice gesture and I was so glad to have made more than enough cookies for them. Isn't it funny how things seem to just work out like that? I mean, were we in sync or what.

SUNDAY, DECEMBER 20, 2009

This and That
Finally out of Bed ...

Yes, I am finally out of bed since treatment on the 10th. Yesterday was actually when I got out of bed and stayed out of bed for most of the day. I did have to lay down 2 different times and catch a nap. I also went to Walmart with my husband and had to sit down twice. Maybe that was pushing it a bit. To be in bed for literally 10 days, one does tend to get cabin fever. I am doing my best to stay down and not over do it before my next treatment on the 31st. Yes, New Years Eve I will be celebrating with a chemo cocktail. Hey I am just glad I am on schedule and staying that way, besides my insurance deductible starts all over Jan 1, so it is best to get as much as possible done this year. That way we will only have 2 treatments for next year to wrangle with financially.

Vision
While I may be getting some good insight through this and having visions, my literal vision is worsening or seems to be. It is very hard to focus and I feel at a loss if I do not have my glasses. I am definitely going to have to get my eyes checked after this is all over. I have a feeling I will have to get used to wearing glasses all the time. A small price to pay.

Grape Juice works for Me
Yep, with everything I have tried, Grape Juice seems to be the one thing that helps keep me regular. I actually started drinking it because I was

hoping it would help lower my platelets, but found constipation was not an issue this time around, Yippee! Trial and error will eventually get you there. The funny thing is I will probably figure most of this out by the time I am done. Oh well, it keeps my brain stimulated.

Bean Burritos

Did you know an average size bean burrito (pinto beans ~4 Tbsp, 1 med size flour tortilla, 1/8 cup shredded cheese) has 25% the recommended daily allowance of Iron, 14 gms of Protein and Calcium. I knew they were good for you, but just didn't know how good and I do crave them now and then. I have been alternating Cream of Wheat and Special K cereal for breakfast daily because they both provide 45% the recommended daily allowance of Iron. Yep, you guessed it my RBC was down from the last time (which was already considered low), so I am doing what I can to get it back up there. Meanwhile, trying to maintain and improve my WBC which came in at 3.9, can I get a whoop whoop! I was mighty proud of myself as that is only 2 tenths of a point off from the lowest target of 4.1 and up from the 2.8 after my first treatment. I did that by making some of the recipes in the cook book the Dr office gave me, Eating Through Cancer. One of my favorite recipes is the Mini Pizza's. They are so easy. All you need is a can of biscuits for the crust, and if you like your pizza red, tomato sauce, and cheese then what ever toppings you like. My husband likes a red pizza with cheese and pepperoni. I prefer white pizza so I just used olive oil and garlic then topped with cheese, mushrooms and artichoke hearts, Yummy to my tummy!

Posted by Angels & HummingBirds & Fairies & CBear
at 11:16 AM

Our trip to Walmart netted me a new friend. This was one of the few times I chose to wear the wig I had gotten from the American Cancer Society. As we were checking out, the cashier complimented me on my hair style. Being the person I am, I told her it was a wig and I was dealing with breast cancer. She was quite surprised, as she said she would have never guessed I was wearing a wig, much less battling breast cancer. Little did I know she had dealt with breast cancer only a few years before and her hair had grown back very nicely. She went on to share with me that she was cancer free and doing very well. From that moment on, I like to think we had become friends.

WEDNESDAY, DECEMBER 30, 2009

House Cleaning

Back a few months ago, I received an email from someone I met at work, and has become a dear friend. She sent me a link to Cleaning for a Reason www.cleaningforareason.org, which she had received from her mother. It is a non profit organization that provides free professional house cleaning services to people fighting cancer. It is a wonderful program and kudos to Debbie Sardone, President/Founder of Cleaning for a Reason for forming this foundation and all of the agencies that work with it.

I speak from experience as one of the first things I did once I was diagnosed was look into cleaning agencies as I knew keeping up the house would be somewhat taxing for me and my husband. The first agency I thought of was Maids of Honor as they give to the community, which we have experienced firsthand in the past. I thought it was only appropriate to return the favor. On the Maids of Honor website www.

azmaidsofhonor.com I saw the pink breast cancer ribbon stating they donate free services for cancer patients through Cleaning for a Reason, so I clicked on it. I read about the program and called Maids of Honor. They explained what I needed to do to work with them and within a week we made an appointment for Maids of Honor to come out and clean my house. The program provides a once a month cleaning for four months. So far they have been out three times and each time they have done a Great job! Everyone from the owner to the office staff to the cleaning staff have been nothing less than wonderful and enthusiastic about helping us out. They seem to sincerely enjoy helping people and the community.

I strongly suggest anyone dealing with cancer look into this program. It is such a relief and so helpful. They have many agencies that work with them across the United States.

Posted by Angels & HummingBirds & Fairies & CBear
at 2:58 PM

I finally called the makeover number to inquire about getting a makeover. I was directed to call Thunderbird Hospital. I found out the next time they were going to have a class and that it was free. They said it was okay to bring someone with me, so I asked my mother if she was interested. I felt it was a good opportunity to continue our bonding. We went and really did enjoy ourselves. Based on my coloring, they gave me a tote bag of cosmetics, moisturizers, and applicators. Everything had been donated.

They asked for a volunteer to show scarf tying techniques and put makeup on. This meant we had to go to the front of the group and show our bald head. When no one opted to do it, I raised my hand. As I approached the front of the group, I was complimented on how I had tied my scarf. I was then asked to demonstrate how I did it. I explained I evenly wrapped a long scarf around my head and tied it in the back at the nape of my neck, as if it were a ponytail. I then shifted slightly to one side and did a macramé knot all the way to the end. Sometimes I would wear a hat over the scarf also.

They proceeded to take us through some tips for taking care of our skin and applying makeup and gave us some information about picking and wearing a wig. Overall, it was a very nice outing and I believe we learned something new.

WEDNESDAY, DECEMBER 30, 2009

#4 Tomorrow

As of this time tomorrow we will be 2/3 of the way through this, 4 down and 2 to go. All I can say is I will be glad when this is all over and I can get on with things … As my Mom says, "It's a temporary situation." I hold on to that like nobody's business.

I have to admit I am somewhat apprehensive about this next treatment, given the events of the last treatment. I guess it is because I don't know if it was the exhaustion or the cumulative effect that made things so hard on me last time. The problem for me is I could only do something about the exhaustion and I have been real good about staying down. So good, that I am driving myself crazy. Oh, then my laptop computer picked up a bloody virus that all the Lysol in the world cannot cure. Besides that, I have been thinking of all kinds of things I would rather be doing than sitting around. Oh well, it's only temporary. Actually after tomorrow it's only about 8 more weeks. Now that does not sound so bad, does it? Considering we have gotten through nearly 19 weeks since the beginning of this ordeal. Wow, when you put it that way where we are now takes on a whole new view. I probably didn't say that right, but you know what I mean. As always, I am doing what I can to stay positive, as a good attitude is the key to recovery when dealing with any kind of craziness life may throw at you. I am hitting this curve ball right out of the park and it is gonna be a Grand Slam ... It wouldn't be the first time!

Posted by Angels & HummingBirds & Fairies & CBear
at 3:33 PM

During my treatment, I received a call from none other than RJ. I felt busted, but he was celebrating the New Year and had had a few to drink. Whew, that was close! I had to field the call myself because Ric was with Mooki at a doctor's appointment across the street. It took longer than he expected, but he got back just in time for my treatment to end.

WEDNESDAY, JANUARY 6, 2010

Noodles

Yep, that is what my arms and legs feel like anytime I try to do anything with them. Something as simple as putting vegetables on a plate to heat in the microwave, renders my arms limps as noodles. This is the worst side effect yet. It all comes down to muscle weakness. I have yet to be able to walk more than 10 steps without having to stop and take a break. It is frustrating because this is day 6 after my last treatment and I do not feel I am any closer to having a good day.

The upside is that I only have to go through this 2 more times.

I will touch base in a few days, because the noodles are getting limp again …

Posted by Angels & HummingBirds & Fairies & CBear
at 4:11 PM

MONDAY, FEBRUARY 1, 2010

It's been a while

Wow, it has been nearly a month since my last blog. Eeeesh, I gotta tell you, I went from feeling like a noodle to putty. I just put myself in that little plastic container and went to sleep or tried to at least. I have to say hands down the worst part so far has been between the 4th & 5th treatment. Everything from mouth sores to constipation plagued me.

I had to get what they call Magic Mouth for the mouth sores. It can also be known as Miracle Mouth. It does work wonders. Then for the constipation they prescribe a brown cow. A brown cow is 1/2 cup prune juice mixed with 1/4 cup milk of magnesia, another thing that works wonders, but there are some precautions. First you want to take it in the morning as once it goes to work (about 1 hour) it keeps on working for about 36 hours, or at least it did for me. Do not under any circumstances trust a fart. Finally drink lots of fluids and keep drinking them. It really does clear your system out, but is somewhat aggressive. So I would not suggest using it often. For the vomiting I took the anti-nausea drug and drank ginger ale. As far as the noodly feeling, well there just wasn't much I could do for it. I believe it has to do with my RBC being too low (9.8), which they had to give me shot for the low RBC on my 4th & 5th treatment. Yes the shot from the 4th treatment did not bring it up, but it didn't lower it as it came in at 9.8 again. We tried to correct my diet to include more iron, but it didn't seem to work. Or maybe it did because my RBC did not drop.

The first thing I did after my 5th treatment was cry. I had hit a low and was saddened by the fact that it wasn't my last treatment. Honestly speaking, I am really sick of being sick. I don't care if I am bald, out of shape, or that my skin feels like sand paper right now. I just want my energy back and to feel really good. Oh and I would also like to have the strength once again to hold my posture. This is all I could think about after my 5th treatment. Okay, so I took a moment to have a pity party. I am entitled, so long as it does not go on too long.

How am I feeling today … pretty okay. Actually, better than I have felt in a while. I have some energy, enough to prepare my own meals and walk around the block yesterday. I didn't go around the block today, but I will tomorrow. I don't know what all this means, but I hope after my 6th treatment I start feeling better 11 days post, so I can start getting my energy back steadily. I so look forward to walking around the block every day and speeding up each time. I have lost 20 pounds through all this and would like to tune it up, if you know what I mean. I also can't wait until I can taste food the way it should taste. For instance, I made a Caesar salad the usual way and in theory it tasted good, but not when I ate it. It didn't taste bad, it just wasn't quite right. I really really miss spicy foods. Spicy food is such a comfort food for me and not being able to eat it through this has been rough.

It won't be long now, we will once again be on the road to normalcy. I believe after my last treatment, I have to take time to let my immune system rebuild. Then I have to have the port removed, which the Oncologist says I should not have removed before a month after my last treatment. Just in case there are any unforeseen complications with my WBC or RBC counts. Once the port is removed I guess the focus is to get my energy back. From what I have been told by other cancer patients and read, it can be slow going. I am going to try real hard to not expect too much from myself. I am only human after all. Tootaloo!

Posted by Angels & HummingBirds & Fairies & CBear

at 7:22 PM

My Research

One thing that kept my mind off the negative effects of what I was going through was my analytical need to know things. What I needed to know is how the heck did I get breast cancer? What did I do or not do to somehow contract this dreaded disease? You see, once I found out I was not genetically predisposed to this disease, the hunt was on. I am one of those people who chose to learn from the challenges I was faced with. Other than losing Kaity, this was the most life threatening and altering challenge I had faced. I was going to win and win big! Not just for myself, but for my family and all those out there I still have something to offer to through Kaity's Way.

So there I was contemplating, where do I begin? I opened my laptop, which I was very thankful for. It did make things easier in so many ways through that time of my life. It was my 2006 Christmas present from my husband and the kids. It has totally been worth its weight in gold over the years. Early on in this journey, I was using it to play games to keep me entertained and my mind on something other than how sick I was. Unfortunately, I must have zigged when I should have zagged and my trusty laptop got a virus. I went to Fry's Electronics to get it fixed. No matter what it cost, I had to get it fixed, it was my lifeline at times. When I was home alone, it was my best friend. It allowed me to stay up-to-date on certain issues and amused me. The young lady behind the counter was so sweet and took a look at it and told me I could fix it by simultaneously hitting two keys and following directions. I, for the life of me, cannot remember what those two keys were, but it did do the trick. By the way, it is not unusual that I don't remember certain things. My memory was and at times still is, for lack of a better term, poop. It was not something I was going to let bug me. Given all the poison that was pumped inside of me, it is a wonder I have any memories at all. Wouldn't it be great if the not-so-great memories could be wiped out for good? Well, maybe not, since they are what remind us of a decision or choice that was not the greatest. The young lady no doubt, saved us some money and I cannot tell you how much I appreciated her helping us out like that. I hope I was able to adequately relay my appreciation for the tip.

Alrighty then, my trusty laptop was back in working order and actually seemed to be better than ever. My first step was to understand the disease as much as I could, so I googled *invasive ductal carcinoma*. I read what Wikipedia had to say about it along with various other breast cancer websites and Web MD. I learned it was the most common type of breast cancers, with 55 percent of those diagnosed with breast cancer having had this type. The upside is because it is the most common type, chances are that there have been more studies and the prognosis was good if caught early enough. Based on what I had read, I was dealing with stage two leaning towards stage three breast cancer. After reading several definitions of what invasive ductal carcinoma is, I had come to a conclusion. I figured if I understood the issue in the simplest of terms, I could address it. My understanding of cancer, no matter where it is in the body, is a group of cells that have not realized their true life span. In other words, every cell in our body has a plan. They are created for a certain purpose and have defined life spans. They were born to accomplish their task, and then die. Cancer cells don't die; they go rogue, mutate, and join with each other, in some cases, to form a tumor.

Now that I had a pretty good idea of what I was dealing with, I could move forward. So, how was it that cells in my body decided to go rogue and mutate? After all, I am the type of person who believes in natural remedies versus conventional remedies. That is not to say I am completely opposed to conventional medicine. Like all things, it has its place and time. Nonetheless, I thought I was eating a pretty good diet. I ate and drank lots of soy products and tried to make sure I was eating balanced meals. When I felt under the weather, I would reach for the Echinacea instead of the usual conventional remedies. I am a firm believer that since we are organic by nature, organic items will have the best effect on us with little, if any, side effects. Although, as with everything, moderation is the key.

I was about 25 to 30 pounds overweight and tried to exercise to lose the weight without success. That was partly because I allowed certain events that had occurred in my life and my job to overtake me. Between the two, I was extremely stressed out. Since 2006, several life-altering things had taken place. I previously mentioned the two most devastating events: the murder of our 17-year-old daughter, Kaity, and the sudden death of my sister, Lorie, at the young age of 43 years old.

We had also dealt with loss of employment and car accidents— one that took a life and three others which were physically damaging for my mother and Lorie. Then a very dear friend of mine passed away suddenly at the age of 46 from thrombosis. I had talked with her the day before she passed, and she told me she did not think she was going to make it. I pleaded with her that she was going to be fine, but she knew.

My cousin's husband had been diagnosed with cancer and passed away only a few months after the diagnosis. As previously mentioned, my aunt and cousin both battled cancer. My Uncle Bob had been in and out of the hospital due to liver problems. Basically, only a very small portion of his liver functioned. He had end stage liver disease.

Then there was the job. Oh my goodness, you talk about a stressful environment. The manager who hired me in August of 2006 had a good heart but had no personal life and expected those who reported to her to be right there with her. She had hired me to supervise a team; yet when I challenged them, she insisted before I have any further conversations with my team, I had to run them past her first. For crying out loud, the issue with my team was I had given them an assignment that several of them did not do. I simply asked them what about the assignment they did not understand. None of them copped to a misunderstanding. They simply shrugged their shoulders. As if to say they just didn't feel like doing it. So, I let them know they needed to get it done ASAP. I told my boss I would not run every potential conversation with my team by her and if she does not trust me to run the team then I will step down and be done with it. I don't do passive aggressive, not then not ever. I am pretty straight forward. Apparently, this very simple solution intimidated her, and she proceeded to let upper management know I scared her. That's why Heidi was told she would probably want to fire me when she came on board as the new manager. Yes, the one who hired me ended up resigning. Working with Heidi alleviated some of the stress, but there was a reconfiguration of duties and I was put on a special project. This project required some focus and its success determined whether or not a certain very large contract was going to be signed. I loved a good challenge, so I went to town with it, and we succeeded in our efforts. The team kicked butt and was very good to work with. The more we gave the more upper management wanted. We gave them more, more, and more and for our troubles received very little in return. That's how it goes when you work for the man. Business is business and don't take it personally.

We were also constantly reminded that there were patients who depended on us and we needed to get the job done. It was as if they thought we didn't get it. We got it alright; yet, upper management was not willing to staff appropriately to get the job done. Instead, they wanted people working overtime. Overtime was cool if it was optional. Most times it was not; it was mandatory. I didn't know they could do that. Goodness, let people have their lives already. The mentality of 'squeeze as much as you can out of the underlings so the executives and shareholders can make millions and pull down some crazy large bonuses' was insane. When the economy took a downturn, they took full advantage of it. It had become an employer's market and they started squeezing even harder. They were still making money hand-over-fist, signing huge contracts and growing the business, but not letting up on the staff, not a single bit. It was a very manipulative, abusive environment and I was right in the middle of it.

There weren't too many days that I didn't go home from work complaining about one thing or another. Ric would listen to me as

I vented, but I got up and continued to put myself through it, day after day. I always told my kids to go to college and get a degree in something you enjoy no matter how much it pays. Just be happy. The silly thing is that I did not even think about taking my own advice. I made alright money (about $50,000 a year) but I didn't feel I was duly compensated for my service and dedication. There were many other things that factored into the environment as well and they were all things I had no control over.

On a stress thermometer, given everything that had happened in the recent years, the mercury was blowing out the top. When we lost Kaity, our world was completely overturned. In an effort to deal with the loss, we formed Kaity's Way. My sister Lorie coined the name. Yep, she was just that creative, sharp, and smart. We had hit upon something that was needed in the community and Kaity's Way took on a life of its own. Helping others can be very therapeutic and healing, so we had discovered. As of April 2008, I was not only working full-time and then some at the day job, but now I was putting in many hours getting Kaity's Way up and running. This meant, between the two I was putting in 70 to 80 hours a week: 50- 60 for the day job and the rest for Kaity's Way.

As previously mentioned, Lorie was very supportive and helped when she could. Lorie also recognized I needed her to not only be my sister but my friend. Lorie lived with us for about a year. After which she lived with us off and on and, eventually, we cosigned so she could have an apartment of her own. I was concerned about her living alone and was going to let our dog, Sedona, go live with her, but the apartments would not allow certain breeds in the complex and German Shepard was one of them. Lorie really enjoyed having her own place again and was getting on with her life. She had neck surgery the summer of 2008 because she was rear-ended in a car accident and had suffered damage to her neck. In early 2009 she had decided she was going to buy a house and started working with a program to clean up her credit and get things situated. On June 7, 2009, Lorie had stopped by the house. She still had a key, so she let herself in. She found me in the bathroom sticking push pins in the wall to hang my jewelry. She looked really tired, basically worn out. She spoke as if she were half asleep. I told her she looked tired. She said she was, and she was going home to take a nap. We hugged and said we loved each other, and she was gone. That was the last I saw of her alive.

All we know is on the evening of June 8, 2009, Lorie was on her way home from a friend's house and stopped at an Asian market for some tea. That was the last thing she did. It wasn't until 1:00pm on June 9, 2009 that anyone noticed her car had been parked in front of the market and called it in. When the emergency team arrived, they found Lorie unresponsive and her temperature was 109 degrees. She was gone, but from what we understand they tried to bring her back, to no avail.

I had lost one of my very best friends now. What the heck! Once again, my family was completely knocked for a loop. We were all at the hospital trying to understand what happened. There was really no explanation. We had not recovered from losing Kaity, losing Lorie was like adding fuel to a fire.

This next part is going to be a bit vague, because it is not my wish to hurt anyone in the writing of this book. What is said is only to make a point regarding my level of stress and how compounded it was.

I don't completely understand it, but after we lost Lorie, my sisters, brother, mother, nieces, and nephews seemed to have shattered into a million individual pieces. There was a lot of anger towards each other that stemmed from our own internal feelings. Some went their separate ways not to speak or have anything to do with the family for several years. Others suffered in silence. We did not have each other to help with the healing process on any level. It was absolutely devastating and unbelievable how so many in a family could simultaneously just call it quits. Looking back the family I was born into, for as long as I can remember is fractured.

With all that said, you have probably come to the same conclusion I had. Stress is what brought on the breast cancer in me. I had come to realize stress is the number one killer of humans. Stress causes cancer by dropping your immune system. Stress causes high blood pressure and various heart diseases. Stress is not biased. It does not care who you are, what you do, or where you come from.

SUNDAY, FEBRUARY 21, 2010

On the Mend

My last treatment was Feb 11, 2010. I went into it with the attitude let's get this done. I just could not wait to say that was it; I am done, no more kicking me down. Well just before they hooked me up to the IV I went to the bathroom and threw up. I am not sure why other than the fact that psychologically I wanted to get it over with before it started. Maybe it was a pre-emptive strike. I didn't throw up after the treatment, so maybe that's it. Who knows exactly why that happened, but it is over, thank God!

When the treatment was all over we came home and I was wiped out, probably more mentally than anything. It wasn't until I was 6 days post that I took the major energy dive. Don't get me wrong I wasn't running laps day 1-5, but I was able to get around without pain or severe fatigue. Day 6 reminded me that there was a toll to be taken before I was on the mend. It hit me like a ton of bricks. I was so frustrated and annoyed at myself. I kind of had a pity party and that annoyed me also. I just couldn't seem to do anything right and being stuck in bed wasn't helping. The previous treatments I hit this energy low phase about day 2 or 3. Since on day 2 or 3 this time around I did not take the energy dive, I thought the energy low was going to be mild. Then KA-BOOM!

Day 7 wasn't any better, but I insisted on lying on the couch instead of staying in the bed. Sometimes when you change the scenery your attitude will change along with it. I believe it helped to some degree, but my energy level was -0-. When I say -0- energy I mean I could not stand for more than 1 minute without feeling like I had to sit down due to pain or fatigue. I know this because I took something from the refrigerator and put it in the microwave for 2 minutes and had to sit down before a minute was up.

Now I am 10 days post and I am feeling better. I feel as if I am finally on the mend. One thing I think helps quite a bit is to take a nice hot as you can take it bath in 1 1/2 cups Epsom salt 3-5 days after your low energy day. I did this after every treatment and each time it did make me feel better in one way or another.

At this point, other than a couple of healing sores in my mouth and a lump in my throat that makes it hard to swallow, I am trying to stay down in an effort to not set myself back. My RBC and WBC were down this last time around, so I really need to make sure I am getting *plenty of iron and vitamins in my diet. My mom is going to come over today and make me some liver (very high in iron), she makes the best liver I have ever tasted. She is also going to make some stuffed peppers to freeze. We are also going to make spanakopita burgers. What are spanakopita burgers you ask? I saw Rachel Ray make them on her show on the food network. It is a simple recipe and looks delicious. It is also figure friendly. I have lost about 23 pounds and really want to keep it off. Anyways, so here is the recipe:*

Ingredients

1/2 red onion

2 garlic cloves

1 1/3 pound ground chicken or turkey

1/2 to 1 cup feta cheese

1 box 10 oz thawed and rung frozen spinach, important you get the moisture out

1 tsp Oregano

Your choice of seasonings to taste (Lawry's, Grill seasoning, sage, rosemary, pepper, salt)

- *Saute the onion and garlic in oil or butter until they become translucent*
- *Put in a large mixing bowl and let cool*
- *To that same bowl add the meat, feta cheese, spinach, oregano, seasonings you prefer and drizzle in some olive oil*
- *Mix it all together and make your patties. Keep in mind the patties are not going to shrink much.*
- *In a large skillet melt some butter (about 2 tbsp) and add olive oil over medium high heat.*

- *Once butter is melted raise the temp to medium high heat and add your patties to the skillet.*
- *If you make just 4 large burgers from this recipe 1" thick you will need to let them cook for no less than 6 minutes on each side.*

If you try this recipe let me know what you think. I am really excited to cook with my mom today. My mom and I share a love for savory food, so this should be fun.

Posted by Angels & HummingBirds & Fairies & CBear
at 8:27 AM

What's Next

The month of March is going to be a tying up the loose ends month. I have to see the oncologist again on the 4th. They will run blood tests to see where I am at with my RBC and WBC. I am going to try hard to pump up my diet so these numbers come back in the good range. I really don't want to have any more shots or get some blood transfused. I just want to be done.

The oncologist will also give me a prescription for some medication I will need to be on for the next 5 years. I am wondering why not just have your ovaries removed instead of taking medication. From what I understand the medication I will be prescribed is supposed to bind to estrogen receptors so cancer cells cannot. Well since estrogen comes from the ovaries, why not just get rid of them. I am going to ask my doctor about this. I will also need to see my regular doctor to get my yearly exam, the eye doctor, and get a mammogram again.

Hopefully, I will have the port removed early in the month also. I can hardly wait until it is gone. It is annoying and I don't like seeing it. I have thrown some ideas at my artist sister for a tattoo to cover the port scar. It's going to be cool. I am hoping she can incorporate bamboo, orchids, hummingbird, angel,s and fairies all around Asian writing meaning Survivor. I can't wait to see what she comes up with.

Posted by Angels & HummingBirds & Fairies & CBear
at 9:34 AM

WEDNESDAY, MARCH 10, 2010

Cleaning Up

On the 4th I saw the oncologist and while I am still anemic, I did not have to get a shot or blood transfused. He just gave me a prescription for folic acid 1mg.

The reason removing the ovaries is not the best solution is they are not the only source of estrogen. From what I understand estrogen also comes from fat cells. So I am on Tamoxifen and so far I am not feeling any side effects. The first day after taking the medication I did have a headache, but that was due to my shoulders being tense, probably from worrying about the side effects. I got so annoyed that I decided I would take it through the weekend and if I had anymore headaches I would call the Doctor on Monday to talk about lowering the dosage. No need to make the call.

I do not have to see the oncologist until July. I am happy about that.

I have to have a mammogram every 6 months on my right breast, so I had that done today. Fortunately, the same person that did my last mammogram did this one. She is a really nice, compassionate person. Getting the mammogram was only slightly uncomfortable. She said the Radiologist was impressed with the surgery and it does not appear an ultrasound is necessary at this time. Music to my ears, I just had to give her a hug and did.

Okay the port comes out on the 18th. The last surgery and I am so glad. It is a 10 minute procedure and is done outpatient at the hospital. I can hardly wait!

Posted by Angels & HummingBirds & Fairies & CBear
at 10:47 AM

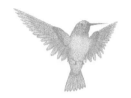

Chapter 16

Getting On With Life

T he March 10, 2010 blog post was the last of them. The port was removed on the 18th and now it's time to get on with it ... it was time to get on with life, to get back in the game. I had finished up all radiation and chemotherapy treatments and as far as I was concerned, I am cancer free! I had completed the full-body, inside-out detoxification and now I was ready to rock and roll. I had a new lease on life and I was going to get all I could out of it. No more holding back on what I wanted to do. I was going to go for it at every opportunity.

As a celebratory escape, Ric and I headed to California for a few days to visit his mother, brother, and my friend, Denise. The first few days we stayed with Ric's mother in Victorville and spent time with her and Cliff. We played games, talked for many hours, went out to dinner, and saw Cliff's new house. It was a very nice relaxing visit. Next, we went to Riverside to spend time with Denise and her family. It was wonderful seeing her three grown daughters, grandsons, son-in-law, mother, and sister. We ate, played rummy, laughed, and talked for hours. It was another wonderful visit, not to mention the weather was beautiful.

Now it was time to get on with the plan for recovery and the business end of life. While sorting out my plan for recovery, we heard from RJ, he would be taking leave in May, which was less than two months away. This made us realize that we needed to discuss how we were going to tell RJ, and Dan for that matter. As always, we decided to be completely honest. We knew there was a chance they would be hurt and scared on some level, but they were reasonable people, so we knew they would understand that we did what we did out of love for them.

Now I needed to get things situated with my employer. Thankfully, I still had a job and Heidi, good to her word, arranged for me to take a position on her team. I returned as an operations supervisor and she worked me in slowly. She understood what chemotherapy did to a person's brain and knew there had been some significant changes since I was last on her team.

When I returned to work, the team was very accepting and compassionate. I could tell they felt for me, and some were uneasy around me. I dealt with this by making light of the situation as often as I could, by cracking jokes and doing silly things to ease the tension. I was bald as a cue ball and at first wore a scarf and/or hat to work. The thing about the hat and scarf was that I was having some difficulty with it shifting on me. While that was a great opportunity to get a good laugh, it got old after a while, so I stopped wearing them and just went au natural.

Going au natural made it so I could get ready within 15 to 20 minutes in the morning. That included showering, makeup, and getting dressed. Maybe it was not such a bad thing after all. I also found some of those little bows in the baby section that had sticky stuff. So, I wore a few of those into work that got a good laugh from time to time. About the April timeframe I started getting peach fuzz on my head. I randomly asked one of the managers who kept his hair really short for a referral to a good barber.

Another order of business was to get back online with Kaity's Way. Strangely enough, after the GYC presentation in October, I did not get a request to present until just after my last treatment. I was so glad for that, because one of the last things I wanted to do was have to decline anyone our services. The other thing to consider was if word of my condition were to get out, people may think that I was going to die and then what would happen to Kaity's Way?

It was not much of a challenge to get back online with Kaity's Way. The requests just started coming in, and the more we accepted, the more requests we received. Heidi, being there when we lost Kaity, was very supportive and understood our mission and as long as I could provide coverage, I was able to take time off to do presentations and set up resource tables. Yes, despite my baldness, I was doing presentations and reaching out to the community on a regular basis. Before I knew it, a path to New York to participate in an event called "It's Time To Talk" had been paved. That is pretty much how it goes with Kaity's Way. There truly is a demand for the service we provide, and word of mouth has been enough to keep us busy.

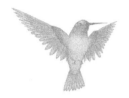

Chapter 17

Time to Come Clean

Before I wrap this up, I wanted to share with you RJ's home coming and how we told him and our son Dan about my cancer. We had to tell them separately. RJ was the first to be told because he came home from Korea on leave in May 2010 before he was to be stationed in Italy. Needless to say, we were very excited. We had not been able to hug him for a little over a year now and so much had happened. I couldn't wait to see him, but I was a little apprehensive about his reaction when he saw me. Only a little because RJ is a great person and he is not one to spend any time assuming anything. He would ask the question if he felt he needed to know. Although, he had been through quite a bit since losing his sister and Aunt Lorie. We were not sure what he had done to work through those losses. Every time we tried to talk with him about Kaity and Lorie, he would change the subject or tell us he would rather not talk about it. Knowing and respecting that everyone grieves in their own way, we left him alone and waited for him to approach us. Thus far, he had not done so. With that in mind, I feared he would lose hope that eventually things would right themselves.

I had a scarf on my head when we saw each other. My hope was that he thought I was just trying a new fashion sense. My gut told me he had a feeling something was off, but he kept to himself about it. Ric and I sat him down and explained my condition and the reason for not telling him. He understood our reasoning and agreed it would have been very difficult for him. He kept a positive attitude as we reassured him that I am cancer free! All was well with RJ; we hugged and had a great time with him before he went to Italy. In case you're wondering, yes, I did go to visit him in Italy for eight wonderful days in April 2011 … another thing I could check off my bucket list …

The conversation with Dan went very well also. We told him during the Thanksgiving vacation we took to Texas with Mooki, her boyfriend, and the baby. We drove 14 hours to Ric's sister Angela's house for Thanksgiving with her, her children, Ric's brother, Cliff, and his Mom. Unbeknownst to us, Ric's brother and mother arranged for Dan to be in Texas for Thanksgiving as well. This was a wonderful and emotional surprise. Dan seemed to be working through his grief and it was apparent he needed to be around this part of his family.

Even though it had been nine months since my last treatment, I still looked a little gaunt. I could tell that the sight of me literally scared my mother-in-law. Try as she might, she was not one to hide her feelings. I understood her fear. Here she has this son who had lost a daughter and I look like I am still on death's door. It was all part of recovery, but not everyone understood that. I figured if my mother-in-law looked that scared, I was sure Dan was somewhat bewildered by my appearance. So, I took him aside one-on-one to delicately explain what had happened and why we chose not to tell him until then. I believe it was a successful conversation as I reassured him that I am cancer free! He gave me a huge hug and was very thankful for being in Texas and that I was okay.

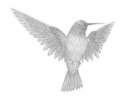

Chapter 18

The Recovery Phase

Whenever I initially started writing this book back in 2010, I thought I would have it published and on the shelves before now. You guessed it life happened. I became very busy and the book was put on the back burner. It became one of those things that I would circle back around to, and I did. Given that I am several years post-cancer, I have realized there is so much more to the recovery phase. I am actually glad I did not finish this book then. It's just another one of those moments, everything happens for a reason.

There are many things that factor into a person's recovery to better health: diet, vitamins, supplements, exercise, mental well-being, and good, knowledgeable, open minded doctors. What I have learned is that each one of those things intertwines with the others. It's a no brainer that a healthy diet and taking vitamins and supplements will lead to good physical health, however it helps to improve mental health as well. Exercise is first thought of to build a person's strength and endurance, yet it also helps to release certain hormones that make us feel better mentally. Good mental health provides us with the positive drive to take care of ourselves. Then there are your doctors to bounce ideas off of, ask questions to, and guide you through recovery.

I pretty much addressed each area with patience, especially when it came to exercise. You see, the chemotherapy had depleted my system so much so that I literally grossed myself out one day. I was simply sitting outside and put the ankle of my right leg on my left knee and saw my calf muscle just drop. I was mortified, but it explained a lot, like the fear in my mother-in-law's face when she saw me in Texas.

Since it was difficult to exercise in the beginning, I looked at the dietary end of my recovery at the same time. With everything intertwining, it only made sense to take a holistic approach to recovery. I also continued to see my doctors on a regular basis.

My first crack at it was to create a check list for myself. Mainly because my memory was so bad, but to also make sure I was doing everything I needed to do for myself daily. The morning list started with exercising, yoga, meditating, eating breakfast, and ended with pooping. Yes, pooping is on my checklist, because as long as I can remember I have never made it a priority to poop. Going through what I had gone through, I found pooping is most definitely a priority and we should make sure we allow time to do so every single day. This morning check list usually takes me about two hours to get through. I am worth it; therefore, the first two hours of every day are mine.

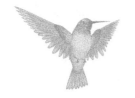

Chapter 19

Diet

As part of my aftercare I was prescribed Tamoxifen, to be taken twice daily. The purpose of the Tamoxifen is to decrease my estrogen levels. Soy contains a natural chemical that mimics estrogen, which is kind of counteractive to the Tamoxifen. Therefore, soy was taken out of my diet. I don't know this for a fact, but it is possible the amount of soy I consumed prior to the diagnosis of breast cancer may have also contributed my condition.

I stay away from white foods such as white flour, sugar, and white rice. They are over-processed and my understanding is that they are just plain not good for you. I guess you might as well eat paper. Oh wait, paper might be better for you due to its fiber content (just kidding)!

My doctor made the following dietary suggestions:

- Eliminate tobacco, alcohol, and sodas
- Eliminate all artificial sweeteners, use stevia sparingly
- Eliminate white sugar and white flour foods
- Eliminate hydrogenated oils, use olive oil instead
- Eliminate milk products, use almond substitute instead
- Eliminate eating/drinking/cooking from plastic containers
- Eat Organic fruits, vegetables, and meats
- Consume a low glycemic diet
- Drink 8 8-ounce glasses of water daily
- Eat gluten free

Under PH Balance and Detoxification, she lists the following to include in my diet:

- Water with organic lemon
- Green powder—Macro Greens, Macro Life with chlorella
- Green vegetables—aloe, asparagus, avocado, broccoli, collard, cilantro, green beans, kale, seaweed, and spinach, just to name a few

She also suggested we get my hormones balanced, which will neutralize estrogen dominance and optimize my thyroid. Avoid xeno and phytoestrogens. Take melatonin nightly if you're not sleeping. I also found on the internet another benefit of Melatonin was it may have cancer fighting properties.[1] Yes, breast cancer is one of the many cancers listed.

I learned on the Dr. Oz show that the following items are considered super foods and it would be a really good thing to incorporate them into your diet:

- Barramundi Fish
- Greens—Fennel, Mustard
- Mangosteen
- Turmeric Tea
- IMO—a Japanese root vegetable

My aunt introduced me to Quinoa, which is also considered a superfood and very versatile. It is actually related to leafy greens like the spinach family. I usually cook up a pot of it and use it in various ways throughout the week. It is so versatile and can be frozen. It can be eaten for breakfast. I make it up the same way I would oatmeal or rice cereal. I add it to salads, beans, sautéed vegetables or use it to create a bed for meat. It has a very mild flavor and goes with most anything you pair it with.

My doctor also suggested the following supplements be added to my daily routine:

- Multivitamin that includes enzymes, amino acids, and minerals
- Omega 3 fatty acids, 2-6 grams
- Vitamin D3, 2,000-5,000 IU
- Vitamin C, 2-4 grams
- Vitamin K, 3 50 mg
- Curcumin, 500 mg

- Selenium, 200 mcg
- Iodine/Iodide, 12.5 mg
- Chlorella, 200 mg
- Resveratrol, 20-100 mg
- Quercetin, 120 mg
- Green Tea Extract, 300 mg

I read a lot of labels to find a way to make sure I was getting the suggested amount of vitamins, minerals, and supplements daily. For instance, instead of taking 300 mg of Green Tea, I drink 24 ounces of good quality green tea a day. I buy it as loose green tea and brew it myself. As for the Chlorella, I drink a green shake. My cousin Susan turned me on to green shakes. My granddaughter drinks them with me and usually gets the lions share, bless her healthy little heart.

I have also learned that incorporating the following items into your regular diet can help to keep cancer at bay.[2]

Garlic	Leeks	Scallions
Brussel Sprouts	Cauliflower	Cabbage
Radishes	Savoy Cabbage	Onion
Turnips	Green Beans	Red Cabbage
Asparagus	Spinach	Beets
Potatoes	Jalapeno Peppers	Red Chicory
Cucumbers	Orange Peppers	Celery

These days, we do not go out to eat very often due to the lack of truly organic restaurants. Therefore, I cook and have learned a new way of doing things since going organic. Actually, I really enjoy cooking and the creativity that comes with it when you choose to follow a certain diet. I also shop at farmers' markets and stores that sell organic items. I stay away from canned goods because many of the cans they are packaged in have a plastic lining that contains BPA. There are some that do not, but that requires you to buy one can and open it to find out if they have the plastic lining.

Basically, when it comes to cooking, I stick with the seasonings we like and incorporate them when I can. I really should start writing things down when I am cooking by the seat of my pants. I have come up with some really great dishes, but they tend to be one-hit-wonders because I don't recall exactly how I managed to put it together. I really love having people over for an organic meal. For some it is the first time and to their surprise it is delicious.

Overall, I've maintained the same diet since 2010, but in 2013 I started having issues with my thyroid. The issues came out of nowhere. All of a sudden, I was sleeping nine to 10 hours a day and had put on five pounds in a matter of two weeks. So, I made an appointment with my family doctor to find out what the heck was going on.

Sure enough, my thyroid had gone nuts. My TSH was 19 (normal is .5 to 4.5/5) and my T4 was nearly nonexistent. TSH causes the thyroid gland to make two hormones: triiodothyronine (T3) and thyroxine (T4). T3 and T4 help control your body's metabolism.[3] So, Houston we have a problem and I was not happy about that. There I was trying so very hard to do everything right with regards to my diet and then this happened. What the heck ... Not to mention, I was wondering if that meant I was going to have to take another medication. No, not me, it wasn't happening. My doctor got the drift and suggested we give it another 30 days to give me some time to do some research and rerun the labs to see where we were at. I asked what I should do in the meantime to not add an additional 10 pounds to my butt as it seemed to be piling on fast. I had been through far too much to gain the weight I lost back. She very simply said, "Go to a plant-based diet." I thought "What the heck? I needed to change my diet yet again by cutting out all meat?" Holy heck, this whole medical issue thing was really beginning to piss me off. So many other people eat what they darn well please, and they seem fine. Yet, I now needed to take on the diet of a rabbit!

Now that I got that out, I realized I had a decision to make: to do or not to do the plant-based diet. Well, given I am a sucker for challenges, challenge accepted! So, for the next 30 days I went cold vegetable (instead of turkey) into a plant-based diet. Mushrooms became my pseudo-meat. Along with a rainbow of vegetables, I ate mushrooms like crazy. I made large amounts of stuffed cabbage, grape leaves, peppers, gluten-free vegetable lasagna, beans, lentils. Yep, I went to town with this and it worked. When I went back to my doctor 30 days later, all my numbers were in check. My doctor literally said, "How did you do this?" I simply told her, "I went to a plant-based diet." She even said, "This is a journal paper." She was so astonished at the results I was able to get, and so quickly, by going to a plant-based diet. I maintained this totally plant-based diet for several more months, but I do allow myself a piece of organic, grass-fed, cage and hormone free meat or fish every now and then. Although most days are totally plant-based, it is nice to have a piece of meat from time to time.

I have to say that the hardest thing for me to stay away from is cheese. It is just so tasty and brings a great flavor to many dishes.

Although, brewer's yeast has helped to curb the amount of cheese I eat. You can use it to make a nacho cheese like condiment for dipping tortilla chips or making mac and cheese. I also put it on salads and add it to dishes because it does have a nice flavor and adds another dimension to the dishes. There are also some pretty good cheese alternatives that are soy as well as dairy free. There is one last thing I want to mention and that is that I have also simplified my green shake when in a pinch ... 4 oz of Georges Aloe Vera Juice (it is truly the best), one tablespoon of organic wheat grass powder, and 4 oz of prune juice ... This helps with digestion, gets you your greens, and moves the pooper. It's good stuff no matter how you look at it and does not taste to bad either.

I know this sounds cliché, but truly everything in moderation in its purest, most organic form is the way to go.

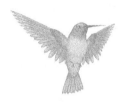

Chapter 20

Mental Well-Being

K nowing what I can and cannot control is the beginning of mental well-being for me. Realizing my limitations and accepting them with an open heart and not seeing them as shortcomings but as messages or guidance to another path. Now, I understand the only control I have is over me and me alone. I have absolutely no control over what someone else does or says, nor am I responsible for what they do or say. I am only responsible for what I do and say and how I choose to perceive things.

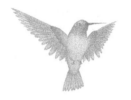

Chapter 21

Within My Control

G iven my research, I now realize I have to decide what I am going to do with the hypothesis that stress is what allowed breast cancer in my life and, therefore, in the lives of my family.

I choose to:

- Abolish stress from my life
- Not to let things I have no control over affect me
- Live happy and enjoy the ones I love
- See the glass as half full.
- Believe everything happens for a reason.
- Allow myself to feel
- Learn from my mistakes

- Appreciate every day
- Not fuss over material things
- Do the things I want to do
- Stop and smell the roses
- Help others in any way I can
- Not to worry about what others think of me since it is really none of my business
- Hold my head high and know I am a wonderful loving person
- Laugh very often
- Love me and make the best of any situation
- Leave my children an inheritance of good memories instead of money

The last one is a kicker ... Well, if you think about it, memories are one of the few things that cannot be taken from you, aside from being stricken with amnesia or going through chemotherapy. Even so, pictures can often fill in the gaps. For my loved ones who have passed, if possible, I ask for a single article of clothing and hold the memories dear. I absolutely love it when I see or smell something that reminds me of the ones I can no longer embrace with affection. Instead, I hug the memory I have of them. When I am missing them more than usual, I will take the article of clothing I have from them, put it up to my face, and take a deep breath to soak in the scent. Oftentimes it will bring me to tears because I miss them so, yet I enjoy the memories I have of them.

While my memory has its challenges due to the chemotherapy, I still have memories creep back from time to time and I will catch myself smiling over a memory I have not thought of in years. It is so heartwarming for me. It is such a great feeling that I want my children to have the same feeling when they think of me after I have left this earthly world.

Since my children are grown, I can be their friend as well as their parent. Therefore, I would rather devote the time now to make more memories with my children and their children. Now this may seem somewhat selfish, but I want to see the joy in their eyes. I want to make them laugh and to laugh with them. I want to experience new things with them. I want them to be proud to call me their mother. I want them to know how much I truly love and adore them. I believe I can do that if they will let me, by giving them life-lasting memories. This brings me wonderful mental health.

One thing my sister Lorie tried to get me to understand were the Four Agreements.[4] Boy was she right. It now makes perfect sense to me.

The Four Agreements are:

1. **Be Impeccable with your Word:** Speak with integrity. Say only what you mean. Avoid using the Word to speak against yourself or to gossip about others. Use the power of your Word in the direction of truth and love.

2. **Don't Take Anything Personally:** Nothing others do is because of you. What others say and do is a projection of their own reality, their own dream. When you are immune to the opinions and actions of others, you won't be the victim of needless suffering.

3. **Don't Make Assumptions:** Find the courage to ask questions and to express what you really want. Communicate with others as clearly as you can to avoid misunderstandings, sadness, and drama. With just this one agreement, you can completely transform your life.

4. **Always Do Your Best:** Your best is going to change from moment to moment; it will be different when you are healthy as opposed to sick. Under any circumstance, simply do your best, and you will avoid self-judgment, self-abuse, and regret.

I sincerely try to live by these agreements every day. Doing so has lifted a great weight off my shoulders.

Once upon a time I was not so impeccable with my words. It wasn't so much that I would gossip. As a matter of fact, I have never liked it when people gossiped and did not mince words when letting them know. I was also very honest, yet not careful with my words in doing so. I was also far too critical of myself and others. I thought it was okay not to expect from anyone else more than yourself, but that is not right. Yet, this was the thought process I was raised with, so for me it was normal. One of the influences in my life felt it was her life mission to always point out what was wrong with something. This left people with the impression that nothing was ever good enough. Although, I truly believe in her eyes, she thought she was helping to make things better by always pointing out the flaws. This general thought process is just wrong, and I found myself doing the same thing to the ones I love. But I don't do that anymore, absolutely not. I have learned to always try to think about what I am going to say and say it not only with integrity but with compassion, understanding, and love. There are also times when saying nothing is more than appropriate and that is when silence is truly golden.

Oh my, taking things personally and making assumptions was second nature to me. If someone was irritable in my presence or short with me, right away I was all over it. I took things very personally, which in turn moved me right into making assumptions. Sometimes I would think to myself: what is their problem, was it something I said or did? Then there were times I would literally straight out say, "What is your issue? Why are you being such and bleep? What is your problem?" There, again, not being impeccable with my words.

Once I came to realize people do have their issues and 99.9 percent of the time they have absolutely nothing to do with me, it was as if the huge chip on my shoulder was removed. I began to stand with self-worth. To take things personally is to take on the issues of many, which is not necessary and incredibly overwhelming. Now with regard to making assumptions ... That was harder nut for me to crack, simply because I am the type of person who likes to solve problems. I will sometimes research or overthink things to death. Once I understood I cannot ever truly get into anyone else's head and know how they feel or what they have been through, it became easy for me not to make assumptions. Therefore, even if I made an assumption, how would I ever know for sure I was right and what the heck does it matter for crying out loud? It is my responsibility to communicate clearly and patiently with others so there are no misunderstandings. Even if there are, usually the person that made the mistake, myself included, was trying to do their best. Either way, assume nothing as it can make a fool out of you at the very least. The flip side to communication is listening whole-heartedly. Listen to hear not respond. Yes, conquering this one agreement will transcend your life; it has done just that for mine.

Since exercising the Four Agreements, I now know 99.9 percent of the time a person's issue will not have anything to do with me because I never do anything to intentionally or unintentionally hurt anyone for any reason. Even when someone has said or done some pretty crappy things to me. I will not let them affect me, because I know in my heart that I am not the cause of their dismay. I always try to do my best and some days I do better than others, but I am so very thankful for each and every day. I am always open ideas and suggestions to better myself for me, the ones I love, and the ones I help.

Here is something that transpired a few years ago that really put my faith in the Four Agreements to the test. Someone asked me via email to not contact them any longer because they did not like the way a mutual friend of ours was treated by me more than a year ago. That was it. This was all the information they gave me. I responded to them via email and apologized they felt that way, but I had absolutely no idea what they were talking about. If I did do something to hurt someone they cared about, I would appreciate knowing what it may have been, otherwise I am unable to make any corrections in my behavior. I never heard back from them again. Now, the old me would have pondered the issue for days on end, making assumptions, wondering what I did. I may have even continued to contact them again and again. I probably would have become angry and personalized it. I may have even sent them an email being less than impeccable with my words, maybe trying to defend myself, all the while just digging a deeper hole for myself, none of which would I have been doing my best.

Nope, I did nothing of the sort. After I responded asking for more information, I left it at that. If I did do something to hurt someone and I reached out to find out what that was, how could I be expected to fix it if I was not let in on what the issue was? I sincerely believe that if someone does something that makes me feel uncomfortable, then I have a responsibility to let them know rather than expect them to read my mind. In instances such as this, it is more than likely a misunderstanding and can be fixed if further discussed. I have never heard from that person or our mutual friend again and I truly do not know if I ever will. Either way, I hold no issues with them and sincerely wish them well.

This, my friends, was truly a test of the Four Agreements and I believe I passed with flying colors. I did not take their words or evasiveness personally. I did not make myself crazy making assumptions trying to figure out what I may have done. I believe I was impeccable with my words and I did my best handling the situation and moved on. Coming to know the Four Agreements has helped me learn there is really only so much I have control over. The extent of my control is me and only me. How I conduct myself is based on the choices I make, and I choose to exercise the Four Agreements to a healthier and happier life.

Other ways I have improved my mental well-being are prayer and meditation, which has been tied in with my yoga practice. I try to meditate and pray every day. Now I am not a religious person, but I am spiritual. Therefore, I do believe in a higher power. I do believe in spirits. I believe our daughter Kaity, my sister Lorie, and the friends and family who have passed on are with me when I need them. Some are there more than others; nonetheless, they are my angels and they guide me every day of my life in all that I say and do. Most times I pray while doing yoga. In circumstances when I am unable to do yoga, I still pray and give thanks for all the answered prayers and blessings.

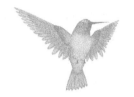

Chapter 22

From Here on Out

After my last treatment in February, I continued to see the oncologist I grew to like every six months like clockwork. My last visit with him was June 2012. I was only a little more than two years post, so why did I stop seeing him? Well, about two months after I saw him in June 2012, I received a letter from my insurance company telling me that he was no longer in their network and I needed to find a new doctor. I've seen this happen before, so I called the doctor's office and asked if the entire office pulled from the network or just my doctor. The receptionist said it was just my doctor because he had suddenly passed away. What the heck! I was taken back. He could not have been much older than me. "How did this happen?" I asked. She explained that about a month after I saw him, he was seeing a patient and excused

167

himself from the room because he felt strange. No sooner did he walk out of the room, he fell to the floor. He had a massive heart attack right there.

Holy crap, what do I do now? I don't know any other oncologists. The receptionist told me my file has been handed over to another doctor in the office. Still in shock, I basically made an appointment to see him the following December, keeping with my every-six-months visits.

Okay folks, this next part is really going to drive home that while doctors are experts in their fields, you—and you alone—are the gatekeeper for your body. Do not under any circumstances let any doctor bully you into taking any medication or doing anything you don't want to do.

I met this new doctor for the first time December 2012. This was after I vetted him on the internet. Nothing spectacular came up, but I did not find any complaints to speak of. At first he seemed like a nice enough guy, but he was not the one. I asked him lots of questions to try to get to know him, but his answers were unremarkable and at times evasive. He told me he literally shared an office with my doctor and was very close to him. Okay, I chilled for a minute, but my gut was not at ease with this guy. The doctor started questioning me about taking Tamoxifen. He wanted to know if I was having any issues with it. I told him no and sometimes I wondered if I were taking a placebo. I was trying to be funny but he didn't see the humor in what I had said. Then he started to discuss another drug with me. He said it had a better success rate, yet he could not articulate why that was. He went on to tell me studies have found that people who have switched to this medication from Tamoxifen have a better chance of living longer.

Then he started talking to me as if I was on death's door. Actually, he was acting like my next step was into my grave, meanwhile talking up this other drug. He really did not explain any side effects and I was not sure if this was because he had not been told this information by the drug rep or if his goal was to get me to switch to this drug. After listening to him for a few minutes, I said, "You can write the prescription, but until I do some research, I will not be filling it." He looked at me as if I had just disrespected him. Who does this guy think he is? God ...

Oh boy, here we go. I hadn't really dealt with any doctors like this since the late 80's when I was a pharmaceutical technician. Most doctors were nice, but there were a few that downright suffered from a hubris complex. How dare a pharmacist question a prescription they had written? Never mind that, at least the pharmacists I worked with were experts in their field and truly cared about the patients they served. It was then that I learned that while doctors do go to school for many years and are very intelligent, they are just as human as I am. They put their pants on one leg at a time and to even act like they are above me or anyone else proves they are only human to think such a foolish thing.

I left the doctor's office thinking that guy just tried to screw with my mind. Yes, I was annoyed and pissed. I called my husband immediately and unloaded the conversation on him. I also called my cousin who is a counselor. Both agreed that this guy was certainly trying to push that drug on me. Something else that came to mind when I was speaking to my husband about the doctor visit was that I am a strong-minded person and can certainly hold my own. Yet, there are others who are, not as strong and assertive as I am. I feel for them in that someone like him could certainly get this over on them simply because they are intimidated by him and his 'doctorness.'

The first order of business when I got home was to get online and check out that drug. Oh my goodness, I could not believe what I found out. That dude was off his rocker if he thought I was going to fill that prescription. From what I read on several different websites and after talking with people, I gathered that drug may help you live a little longer, but your quality of life was poop, to say the least. People had been rendered in wheelchairs due to the side effects it had on the bones and joints. They had no energy, as if the life has been sucked right out of them. Other side effects included weight gain, fuzzy brain, depression ... you name it and someone felt it after starting that drug. I immediately called the doctor's office and left him a message saying I would not take that drug and I would like for him to refill my Tamoxifen. The doctor called me the next day. My message did not require a call from him to me, just him to the pharmacy to refill my Tamoxifen. He apparently didn't listen to my message because he asked me why I had called. I explained to him what I had found online and suggested he look the drug up as well to read the reviews. He reiterated his stance about the drug and said he thought I was making a mistake. I then reiterated I would not take the drug and I would appreciate it if he would call the pharmacy to refill my Tamoxifen prescription, which was done.

Fast-forward six months to my next appointment with him. Yes, I did go see him again, because I had to confirm if it was him or me that day. Maybe I was in a mood. Maybe I took something he said out of context. Who knows, maybe he checked out the reviews I mentioned and came to his senses. The visit started off with the nurse practitioner coming in as she was reviewing my chart. Introductions were made because I had never met her. After further review of my chart she said, "So you are not taking any medication?" Aw man, did it really say that in my chart? I looked at her and said, "I am on Tamoxifen. The doctor called in the refill after my last visit." I went on to explain the conversation the doctor and I had about the other drug and how I refused to take it. With a very serious look on her face she said, "Well, the doctor is not going to like this." I looked at her like, what did you just say to me and responded with, "Be that as it may, I am in charge of this body and I will decide what goes in it." She was taken back by my response and probably the look on my face, because no doubt she got the Guinn look. This is what we refer to as our family stink eye. Who the heck did she think she was talking to? I was not intimidated by the doctor or her for that matter. I cannot even tell you how annoyed I was at that moment. She left the room to retrieve the doctor. I then started counseling myself to breathe and calm down. No stress, no stress, no stress.

Now, it was the doctor's turn as if they were a tag team. He came in and was cordial to begin with, but eventually launched into why I should take the other drug instead of Tamoxifen. Again, I mentioned the reviews to him and that I preferred quality rather than quantity of life. He then asked me what I did for a living. Huh, what does that have to do with any of this? But I play along. I told him that I ran a non-profit organization, which, for whatever reason, rendered him speechless for a moment. Then he asked me if I get my annual well woman checks ups. I told him I did. He said, "That was good because one percent of women who took

Tamoxifen had gotten cancer of that area." Seriously! Was he of the mind there was no way I could fall into the 99 percent who do not? Okay, that did it. I was done with this dude. I had absolutely had it with him and his negative attitude. It was not me, it was him. He told me again I was making a mistake, for which I said, once again, with a bit more force and the Guinn look maxed out, "Be that as it may, I am in charge of this body and I will decide what goes in it!" He then instructed the nurse practitioner to write a prescription for Tamoxifen and I was on my way. That was the last time for me. They asked if I wanted to schedule my next appointment I declined, paid my co-pay and left. Goodbye, sayonara, adios, I was out of there, never to return. As I approached my car, I wondered if that dude had stock in the company or something. Darn it, I wished I would have thought of that while I was in his office. Lorie certainly would have with her witty mind.

You are probably wondering what drug I was talking about. Well, I have withheld the name because I am hoping this book will teach people to research, research, research … What you put or do not put in your body is your choice and no one else's when you get right down to it. So, if you don't do your research, you need to be prepared to accept some of the responsibility for any negative outcomes. Just because someone with letters and such behind their name says it is so, doesn't necessarily mean it is so.

My next step was to find a doctor who had an open mind and would treat me like I was going to live, a doctor who was hopeful and preferred to take a holistic approach. I needed a doctor who did not resort to bullying or intimidation. I needed a doctor who cared about me as a living person.

I came up empty with anyone who took my insurance. Financially, we cannot come out of pocket for very much since I went full-time with Kaity's Way. The reason being was I took a 70 percent cut in pay, but it was doing that or not accomplish our mission. There were too many young people out there craving our message to deny them. I even asked my family doctor if she knew of an oncologist who would fit the bill. She did not. Little did I know she was standing right in front of me less the oncologist part. There she was, right under my nose the whole time. Isn't that just how it works? I asked her to take over my care regarding the breast cancer. She said she would but was very clear in that she did things differently and it was important I understood that. We talked about the plan. The first order of business was to get off the Tamoxifen, which was music to my ears. By now I had taken it for nearly four years without issue, but I have read a lot of books that support alternative methods to keep diseases such as cancer out of one's life. One such alternative is mushrooms. Awesome, I love mushrooms. She knew I researched everything, so she gave me some information about a mushroom supplement as well as another alternative that included turmeric. Early on, I mentioned several other changes I made with regard to the cancer and my thyroid. I also read the books and checked out the videos she suggested. I switched out the Tamoxifen for the mushroom and turmeric supplements. Mushrooms are absolutely fascinating when it comes to their healing properties. They are certainly worth looking into.

My hair growing back has been a slow process but it's getting there nonetheless. I have a lot of fun with the hair I do have. We get creative with color, cuts and styling. Heck it's only hair, it will grow back. Kelly, Rj's fiancé is now doing my hair. This gave us a great opportunity to bond and we did just that. We have become very close and she is nothing less than a daughter to us.

I continue to do my self-breast exams the first day of every month. I have a reminder that hangs in the shower. It has become a habit, so I hardly see the reminder any more.

I mentioned my Bucket list earlier. Well, here is what I have so far, and I do keep adding to it:

- ✓ Sky diving
- ✓ Go to the Lion's Den in Pinetop
- ✓ Parasailing
- ✓ Go to Italy
- ✓ Take a Cruise
- ✓ Zip line
- ✓ Remodel my house
- ✓ Spend time with horses
- • Take a family vacation with all our children and their children
- • Vacation in Bali or Bora Bora

You may have noticed there are two on my bucket list that are not with a check mark. They are the most expensive of all and ones that I will do someday, once I get the funds. Currently, I have placed a large jar in my living room. I use it to collect change for the family vacation. I have let the kids know that is what it is for and they put their coins in it when they come over to visit. We collect our coins and save them for the grandkids, because they love to make deposits into the jar.

As I mentioned, I have read several books about cancer. I have to say the one book that really got my attention is called *KnockOut* by Suzanne Somers. She interviewed several specialists and doctors in the field. They addressed the many aspects of cancers and the various methods to address and/or cure one of cancer. It is certainly worth the read before making any decisions about treatment.

In closing, I believe there are many who can be helped by *C is for Conquer*: people dealing with a cancer diagnosis, those that support them, and practitioners. It is my sincere hope that this book has helped you or someone you know in one way or another. If nothing else, I hope you found it encouraging and empowering, not to mention gave you a good laugh every so often.

About the Author

Bobbi Sudberry is a native Arizonan, born in Ajo, Arizona to a family of copper miners. In the seventh grade she wrote a paper about aliens. It was so well written she was asked to go to the younger grade classes to read the story to the students. Life happened, so Bobbi dropped the pen, but not forever. In her 40s, she realized she had never lost her ability to put pen to paper and began writing again. Only this time, she is sharing one of her own true stories. Bobbi has been on many journeys, some of her choosing, some not so much. Nonetheless, every trial and tribulation she has experienced she chooses to look at as life lessons. She has a sincere want to help others and hopes the sharing of her journey will provide comfort and a chuckle for others to brighten their day. Bobbi is the mother of five children and lives in Phoenix, Arizona with her husband, Ric, and Simba and Xena, their canine children.

Reference

1 http://www.lef.org/magazine/mag2007/jun2007_nu_melatonin_01.htm

2 *Anti-Cancer A New Way of Life, by David Servan-Schreiber, MD, PhD*

3 http://www.webmd.com/women/thyroid-stimulating-hormone-tsh

4 http://www.toltecspirit.com/

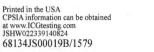